Complex Regional Pain Syndrome

What Do I Do Now?—Pain Medicine

SERIES EDITORS

Mark P. Jensen and Lynn R. Webster

PUBLISHED AND FORTHCOMING TITLES:

Complex Regional Pain Syndrome

Edited by

Jijun Xu, MD, PhD

Associate professor of Anesthesiology

Department of Pain Management

Department of Inflammation and Immunity

Cleveland Clinic Lerner College of Medicine

Case Western Reserve University

Lynn R. Webster, MD

Executive Vice President, Scientific Affairs

Dr. Vince Clinical Research

Overland Park, KS, USA

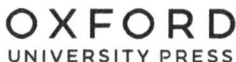

OXFORD
UNIVERSITY PRESS

OXFORD
UNIVERSITY PRESS

Oxford University Press is a department of the University of Oxford.
It furthers the University's objective of excellence in research, scholarship,
and education by publishing worldwide. Oxford is a registered trade mark of
Oxford University Press in the UK and certain other countries.

Published in the United States of America by Oxford University Press
198 Madison Avenue, New York, NY 10016, United States of America.

CIP data is on file at the Library of Congress

This material is not intended to be, and should not be considered, a substitute for medical or other
professional advice. Treatment for the conditions described in this material is highly dependent on
the individual circumstances. And, while this material is designed to offer accurate information with
respect to the subject matter covered and to be current as of the time it was written, research and
knowledge about medical and health issues is constantly evolving and dose schedules for medications
are being revised continually, with new side effects recognized and accounted for regularly. Readers
must therefore always check the product information and clinical procedures with the most up-to-date
published product information and data sheets provided by the manufacturers and the most recent
codes of conduct and safety regulation. The publisher and the authors make no representations or
warranties to readers, express or implied, as to the accuracy or completeness of this material. Without
limiting the foregoing, the publisher and the authors make no representations or warranties as to the
accuracy or efficacy of the drug dosages mentioned in the material. The authors and the publisher do
not accept, and expressly disclaim, any responsibility for any liability, loss, or risk that may be claimed
or incurred as a consequence of the use and/or application of any of the contents of this material.

ISBN 978–0–19–764069–2

DOI: 10.1093/med/9780197640692.001.0001

Printed by Integrated Books International, United States of America

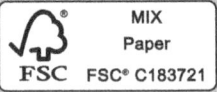

Contents

Preface

CRPS: WHAT DO I DO NOW?

Complex regional pain syndrome (CRPS) is a perplexing and often debilitating condition that challenges both patients and healthcare providers alike. It can emerge unexpectedly following injuries, medical procedures, or trauma, casting a shadow of unrelenting pain and inflammation over the lives of those affected. Although CRPS can manifest in various parts of the body, it most commonly afflicts the arms, legs, hands, or feet. In the ever-evolving landscape of medical knowledge, our understanding of CRPS continues to advance, shedding new light on its complexities and potential treatment strategies.

The management of CRPS demands not only clinical expertise but also a deep understanding of its multifaceted nature. Each case presents unique challenges, and staying up to date with the latest developments in CRPS is essential for providing effective care.

CRPS: What Do I Do Now is a comprehensive guide designed to equip healthcare professionals, students, and anyone interested in understanding and managing CRPS with the knowledge and tools needed to navigate this intricate condition. Within these pages, we present a collection of 13 high-yield clinical cases that encompass a broad spectrum of CRPS-related topics. These cases delve into crucial aspects of CRPS, including its epidemiology, diagnosis, differential diagnoses, pathophysiology, conventional and interventional management, choices of neuromodulation, ketamine infusion therapy, strategies for prevention, CRPS in pediatric patients, and exploration of adjuvant and emerging therapies.

Our highly focused discussions aim to keep readers abreast of the latest updates and breakthroughs in CRPS research and treatment. By consulting this volume, you will gain the knowledge and confidence needed to formulate a contemporary plan for managing this devastating pain syndrome effectively.

CRPS: What Do I Do Now serves as an ideal pocket guide for those seeking a concise yet comprehensive resource to help them navigate the essentials and advancements necessary for CRPS management. We hope that this volume empowers you to face the challenges posed by CRPS with greater insight, empathy, and clinical acumen, ultimately improving the lives of individuals grappling with this enigmatic condition.

With the guidance provided within these pages, we invite you to embark on a journey toward a deeper understanding of CRPS and the development of more effective approaches to its management. Thank you for joining us in our mission to illuminate the path forward in the realm of CRPS care.

—Jijun Xu, MD, PhD
—Lynn Webster, MD

Contributors

Salahadin Abdi, MD, PhD
Department of Pain Management
University of Texas, MD Anderson
Cancer Center
Houston, TX, USA

Magdalena Anitescu, MD, PhD
Department of Pain
Management
University of Chicago
Chicago, IL, USA

Youstina Bolok, MS-IV
Department of Pain
Management
Cleveland Clinic
Cleveland, OH, USA

Jianguo Cheng, MD, PhD
Department of Pain Management
and Neurosciences
Cleveland Clinic
Cleveland, OH, USA

Mark A. Chmiela, MD
Staff Physician
Velazquez Pain Relief Center
Las Vegas, NV, USA

Corinne Cooley, DPT, OCS
Division of Pain Medicine
Stanford Medicine
Stanford, CA, USA

Shrif Costandi, MD
Department of Pain Management
Cleveland Clinic
Cleveland, OH, USA

Jagan Devarajan, MD
Department of Pain Management
Cleveland Clinic
Cleveland, OH, USA

Kerolous Eldeeb, MS-I
Department of Pain Management
Cleveland Clinic
Cleveland, OH, USA

Alexander Foster, MD
Department of Pain
Management
University of Chicago
Chicago, IL, USA

Cyrus Ghaffari, MD
Department of Physical Medicine
and Rehabilitation
Stanford University School of
Medicine
Stanford, CA, USA

Justin C. Grubbs, MD
Department of Anesthesiology and
Perioperative Care
University of California
San Francisco, CA, USA

Brittney Jones, PsyD
Division of Pain Medicine
Stanford Medicine
Stanford, CA, USA

Jonathan W. Kim, MD
Department of Anesthesiology
David Grant US Air Force
Medical Center
Fairfield, CA, USA

Michael Leong, MD
Division of Pain Medicine
Stanford Medicine
Stanford, CA, USA

Steven Mach, MD
Department of Pain Management
University of Texas, MD Anderson
Cancer Center
Houston, TX, USA

Beth Minzter, MD
Department of Pain Management
Cleveland Clinic
Cleveland, OH, USA

Emily Moore, PhD
Division of Pain Medicine
Stanford Medicine
Stanford, CA, USA

Lawrence R. Poree, MD, MPH, PhD
Department of Anesthesiology and
Perioperative Care
University of California
San Francisco, CA, USA

Richard W. Rosenquist, MD
Department of Pain Management
Cleveland Clinic
Cleveland, OH, USA

Vafi Salmasi, MD
Department of Anesthesiology,
Perioperative and Pain Medicine
Stanford University School of
Medicine
Stanford, CA, USA

Samuel Samuel, MD
Department of Pain Management
Cleveland Clinic
Cleveland, OH, USA

Sajan Shah, MD, MBA
Department of Anesthesiology,
Perioperative and Pain Medicine
Stanford Health Care
Stanford, CA, USA

Shiqian Shen, MD, PhD
Center for Translational Pain
Research
Massachusetts General Hospital/
Harvard Medical School
Boston, MA, USA

David D. Sherry, MD
Professor of Pediatrics,
Emeritus
Children's Hospital of
Philadelphia
Perelman School of Medicine at the
University of Pennsylvania
Philadelphia, PA, USA

Zhuo Sun, MD
Department of Anesthesiology
Augusta University
Augusta, GA, USA

Pavan Tankha, MD
Center for Comprehensive Pain
Recovery
Cleveland Clinic
Cleveland, OH, USA

Vivianne L. Tawfik, MD, PhD
Department of Anesthesiology,
Perioperative and Pain
Medicine
Stanford University School of
Medicine
Stanford, CA, USA

Oluwatoyin Thompson, MD
Department of Anesthesiology
Emory University School of
Medicine
Atlanta, GA, USA

**Allie Van Nuys, OTR/L,
OTD, CLT**
Division of Pain Medicine
Stanford Medicine
Stanford, CA, USA

Amy Wang, MD
Department of Anesthesiology,
Perioperative and Pain Medicine
Stanford University School of
Medicine
Stanford, CA, USA

Wenbao Wang, MD
Department of Physical Medicine
and Rehabilitation
Baylor University Scott & White
Waxahachie, TX, USA

**Anna Woodbury, MD,
MSCR, C.Ac**
Department of Anesthesiology
Emory University School of Medicine
Atlanta, GA, USA

Jijun Xu, MD, PhD
Associate professor of Anesthesiology
Department of Pain Management
Department of Inflammation and
Immunity
Cleveland Clinic Lerner College of
Medicine
Case Western Reserve University

Yan Yin, MD
Department of Pain Management
West China Hospital
Chengdu, Sichuan, China

1 The Origin

Amy Wang, Cyrus Ghaffari, Vafi Salmasi, and Vivianne L. Tawfik

Case

A 65-year-old woman complains of a painful left upper
extremity. She reports fracturing her left wrist in a
fall 2 months ago, and she wore a cast for 4 weeks.
She also recalls her cast feeling uncomfortably
tight during that time. Her past medical history
includes hypertension (for which she takes lisinopril
daily), migraines, and depression. She has an aunt
who was diagnosed with complex regional pain
syndrome (CRPS) 2 years ago. Examination shows
an edematous, erythematous, and warm left hand
with thickened nails. Last week, she received her first
COVID vaccination.

What Do I Do Now?

EPIDEMIOLOGY

The incidence of complex regional pain syndrome (CRPS) has been investigated by multiple retrospective population-based studies. Incidences have ranged from 5.5 to 26.2 per 100,000 person-years.[1,2] The Sandroni study found the incidence rate of CRPS type I, defined as CRPS without known nerve injury, was 5.46 per 100,000 person-years, and the incidence rate of CRPS type II, defined as CRPS with known nerve injury, was 0.82 per 100,000 person-years. CRPS is more commonly seen in women with a female-to-male ratio ranging from 2:1 to 4:1.[1] Some studies found that females are up to three times more likely than males to have CRPS, as seen in the de Mos study,[2] with a ratio of 3.4:1. Another nonmodifiable risk factor is age, with the highest incidence seen in women between the ages of 61 and 70.[2] In a large retrospective cohort of 1,043 patients with CRPS, the most common inciting events were fractures (44%), blunt traumatic injuries including sprains (21%), surgery (12%), and carpal tunnel syndrome (7%).[3] Johnson et al.[4] found that, in their initial cohort of CRPS patients, CRPS type I was more prevalent than CRPS type II (89% vs. 11%). After evaluation with magnetic resonance neurography, a novel technique that has high contrast and spatial resolution to better visualize peripheral nerves, CRPS type I was less prevalent than CRPS type II (27% vs. 73%). This study shows the challenges of accurately categorizing CRPS and the need to adopt approaches with higher specificity.

RISK FACTORS

Injuries

In our case, the patient reports fracturing her left wrist in a fall. Fractures, sprains, and elective surgeries have been associated with a higher risk of developing CRPS. Spontaneous onset is uncommon.[2] In a cohort of 1,549 patients with wrist fracture treated nonsurgically, the incidence of CRPS was 3.8% at 4 months. In this cohort, having a pain score of 5 or greater was correlated with the development of CRPS.

Immobilization or Cast Tightness

Our case study patient wore a cast for 4 weeks. She also recalls her cast feeling uncomfortably tight during that time. Managing bone fractures with immobilization and cast tightness have been suggested as risk factors for CRPS. Pepper et al.[5] found that healthy human volunteers undergoing immobilization had mild signs of CRPS (cold and mechanical hypersensitivity). Possible factors include the prolonged disuse of the affected limb and deprivation of sensory input (National Institutes of Health fact sheet). Evidence that fracture, immobilization, and casting result in the expression of inflammatory mediators and CRPS changes (allodynia, warmth, and edema) has also been shown in rodent models.[6,7]

Medications and Medical Conditions

Our patient's past medical history includes hypertension (for which she takes lisinopril daily), migraines.Several studies have evaluated the relationship between the development of CRPS and various medications and medical conditions. In a population-based, case-control study, de Mos et al. found that the use of angiotensin-converting enzyme (ACE) inhibitors at the time of trauma was associated with increased risk of CRPS.[8] Interestingly, both long-term use and high doses had stronger associations with CRPS. This dose-dependent effect provides further evidence supporting a link between ACE inhibitors and CRPS. A potential mechanism may be decreased degradation of ACE-dependent substance P and bradykinin, leading to increased neurogenic inflammation.[9,10]

Other significant risk factors noted by de Mos et al. include migraine, osteoporosis, and use of nonsteroidal anti-inflammatory drugs. A cross-sectional study in 2010 supported de Mos et al.'s findings that migraine is associated with CRPS, whereas nonmigraine headaches are not.[11] Patients with CRPS were 3.6 times more likely to have migraine than the general population. Mean age of onset of CRPS was earlier in those with migraine (34.9 ± 11.1 years) compared with those without (46.8 ± 14.9 years). In addition, more extremities were affected by CRPS in patients with migraine compared with those without headaches or those with tension-type headaches. Both central sensitization and neurogenic inflammation play significant roles in migraine and CRPS, which may explain the pathophysiologic connection between the two disorders.[11]

Psychological Factors

Our patient's past medical history includes depression. It is widely accepted that the perception of pain, both acute and chronic, is closely intertwined with psychological factors. However, there is no evidence that psychological factors increase risk for the development of CRPS. de Mos et al.'s population-based case-control study found that psychological factors were not associated with CRPS onset.[8] A prospective multicenter study of 569 patients with a single fracture analyzed multiple psychological factors—depression, somatization, agoraphobia, insufficiency, interpersonal sensitivity, insomnia, and life events—none of which predicted the development of CRPS type I.[12] A systematic review concluded that while CRPS is associated with both negative psychological outcomes (e.g., increased depression and anxiety) and negative psychosocial outcomes (e.g., reduced quality of life, impaired occupational function), research does not support specific personality or psychopathological predictors of developing CRPS.[13] However, in patients with CRPS, psychological and behavioral factors can exacerbate pain and dysfunction, making psychological evaluation followed by cognitive-behavioral pain management treatment beneficial in the effective management of chronic CRPS.[14] A cross-sectional study of patients with CRPS or low back pain showed a stronger association between pain severity and disability with psychological factors in CRPS compared with low back pain.[15] Altogether, the literature seems to suggest that while psychological factors may not be a risk factor for developing CRPS, they play a role in the disease course of existing CRPS.

Genetics

Our patient has an aunt who was diagnosed with CRPS 2 years ago. Early case reports describing familial clusters of early-onset CRPS suggested a potential genetic component.[16] Mailis and Wade first described certain alleles of the human leukocyte antigen (HLA) system as susceptibility factors for

CRPS.[17] A Dutch study looking at 31 families with two or more relatives with CRPS found that patients with familial CRPS expressed a more severe phenotype, as described by younger age of onset, multiple affected extremities, and presence of dystonia.[16] Despite research identifying leukocyte antigen polymorphisms, tumor necrosis factor-α polymorphisms, and even distinct DNA methylation profiles associated with CRPS, no studies observed a clear inheritance pattern.[18–20] More studies are needed to determine if and how genetic factors play a role in the development of CRPS.

Post-Vaccination

Our patient received her first COVID vaccine last week. Whether vaccination is a risk factor for CRPS is an important topic, especially given the rise in anti-vaccine sentiments rooted in misinformation and the age of social media. There is currently no scientific evidence of association between vaccination and the subsequent development of CRPS. In June 2013, after highly publicized media reports in Japan alleged an association between HPV vaccination and CRPS after the publication of a small case series,[21] the Japanese Ministry of Health, Labor, and Welfare temporarily suspended its national HPV vaccination recommendation.[22] The fear brought on by these claims, followed by the gravity of the government's suspension, led to global spread of the news, prompting research to evaluate whether an association between HPV vaccination and CRPS truly existed. Huygen et al. conducted an independent analysis of all possible HPV vaccine-associated cases of CRPS and found that the observed rate of CRPS after vaccination was in fact significantly lower than would be expected by chance in this demographic group.[23] The researchers thus concluded that there was insufficient evidence to suggest an association between the HPV 16/18 vaccination and CRPS. A follow-up study conducted by US Centers for Disease Control and Prevention researchers used the Vaccine Adverse Event Reporting System (VAERS) to evaluate how US-reported data compared to the Huygen et al. study.[24] Searching for primary reports of CRPS reported to VAERS after any HPV vaccine, Weinbaum and Cano identified that CRPS reports made up 0.07% of adverse event reports. They noted that a small number of CRPS cases have been reported following other injectable vaccines and may have resulted from minor trauma from the injection or improper injection technique.[25] Finally, there is just one published report of transient worsening of symptoms in patients with known CRPS type I after mRNA-based COVID-19 vaccination. In these three CRPS patients, acute clinical worsening after vaccination was transient and effectively managed with adjustment of each patient's individualized therapy.[26] There are, however, multiple mechanisms through which viral infection, such as by SARS-CoV2 (COVID-19) infection may contribute to nociceptor sensitization and therefore exacerbate existing pain states.[27] In conclusion, with monitoring and guidance by their physicians, CRPS patients should not be precluded from safely following vaccination guidelines, especially given the risks associated with COVID-19 infection, not only systemically, but also regarding aggravating existing pain conditions. How the emerging condition of "long COVID" may also affect patients with CRPS remains unknown.

KEY POINTS TO REMEMBER

- Complex regional pain syndrome (CRPS) has a higher prevalence in females.
- CRPS is most often triggered by fractures, sprains, or minor surgery and is rarely spontaneous.
- Immobilization and the perception of cast "tightness" are risk factors for the development of CRPS.
- A history of migraines and the use of angiotensin-converting enzyme (ACE) inhibitors have been associated with the development of CRPS.
- Psychological factors do not seem to predispose to CRPS; however, they can exacerbate the disease course and should be considered in the development of a multidisciplinary treatment plan.
- Vaccination does not appear to cause CRPS, but viral illness may exacerbate CRPS symptoms.

Suggested Reading

Bean DJ, Johnson MH, Kydd RR. Relationships between psychological factors, pain, and disability in complex regional pain syndrome and low back pain. *Clin J Pain*. 2014;30(8):647–653.

de Mos M, de Bruijn AG, Huygen FJ, Dieleman JP, Stricker BH, Sturkenboom MC. The incidence of complex regional pain syndrome: A population-based study. *Pain*. 2007;129(1–2):12–20.

Ott S, Maihofner C. Signs and symptoms in 1,043 patients with complex regional pain syndrome. *J Pain*. 2018;19(6):599–611.

References

1. Sandroni P, Benrud-Larson LM, McClelland RL, Low PA. Complex regional pain syndrome type I: Incidence and prevalence in Olmsted county, a population-based study. *Pain*. 2003;103(1–2):199–207. doi:10.1016/s0304-3959(03)00065-4

2. de Mos M, de Bruijn AG, Huygen FJ, Dieleman JP, Stricker BH, Sturkenboom MC. The incidence of complex regional pain syndrome: A population-based study. *Pain*. 2007;129(1–2):12–20. doi:10.1016/j.pain.2006.09.008

3. Ott S, Maihofner C. Signs and symptoms in 1,043 patients with complex regional pain syndrome. *J Pain*. 2018;19(6):599–611. doi:10.1016/j.jpain.2018.01.004

4. Johnson EM, Yoon D, Biswal S, Curtin C, Fox P, Wilson TJ, et al. Characteristics of patients with complex limb pain evaluated through an interdisciplinary approach utilizing magnetic resonance neurography. *Front Pain Res*. 2021;2(11). doi:10.3389/fpain.2021.689402

5. Pepper A, Li W, Kingery WS, Angst MS, Curtin CM, Clark JD. Changes resembling complex regional pain syndrome following surgery and immobilization. *J Pain*. 2013;14(5):516–524. doi:10.1016/j.jpain.2013.01.004

6. Birklein F, Ibrahim A, Schlereth T, Kingery WS. The rodent tibia fracture model: A critical review and comparison with the complex regional pain syndrome literature. *J Pain*. 2018;19(10):1102 e1101–1102 e1119. doi:10.1016/j.jpain.2018.03.018

7. Cropper HC, Johnson EM, Haight ES, Cordonnier SA, Chaney AM, Forman TE, et al. Longitudinal translocator protein-18 kDa-positron emission tomography imaging of peripheral and central myeloid cells in a mouse model of complex regional pain syndrome. *Pain*. 2019;160(9):2136–2148. doi:10.1097/j.pain.0000000000001607

8. de Mos M, Huygen FJ, Dieleman JP, Koopman JS, Stricker BH, Sturkenboom MC. Medical history and the onset of complex regional pain syndrome (CRPS). *Pain*. 2008;139(2):458–466. doi:10.1016/j.pain.2008.07.002

9. Blair SJ, Chinthagada M, Hoppenstehdt D, Kijowski R, Fareed J. Role of neuropeptides in pathogenesis of reflex sympathetic dystrophy. *Acta Orthop Belg*. 1998;64(4):448–451. https://www.ncbi.nlm.nih.gov/pubmed/9922551

10. Skidgel RA, Erdos EG. Angiotensin converting enzyme (ACE) and neprilysin hydrolyze neuropeptides: A brief history, the beginning and follow-ups to early studies. *Peptides*. 2004;25(3):521–525. doi:10.1016/j.peptides.2003.12.010

11. Peterlin BL, Rosso AL, Nair S, Young WB, Schwartzman RJ. Migraine may be a risk factor for the development of complex regional pain syndrome. *Cephalalgia*. 2010;30(2):214–223. doi:10.1111/j.1468-2982.2009.01916.x

12. Beerthuizen A, Stronks DL, Huygen FJ, Passchier J, Klein J, Spijker AV. The association between psychological factors and the development of complex regional pain syndrome type 1 (CRPS1): A prospective multicenter study. *Eur J Pain*. 2011;15(9):971–975. doi:10.1016/j.ejpain.2011.02.008

13. Lohnberg JA, Altmaier EM. A review of psychosocial factors in complex regional pain syndrome. *J Clin Psychol Med Settings*. 2013;20(2):247–254. doi:10.1007/s10880-012-9322-3

14. Bruehl S, Chung OY. Psychological and behavioral aspects of complex regional pain syndrome management. *Clin J Pain*. 2006; 22(5):430–437. doi:10.1097/01.ajp.0000194282.82002.79

15. Bean DJ, Johnson MH, Kydd RR. Relationships between psychological factors, pain, and disability in complex regional pain syndrome and low back pain. *Clin J Pain*. 2014;30(8):647–653. doi:10.1097/AJP.0000000000000007

16. de Rooij AM, de Mos M, Sturkenboom MC, Marinus J, van den Maagdenberg AM, van Hilten JJ. Familial occurrence of complex regional pain syndrome. *Eur J Pain*. 2009;13(2):171–177. doi:10.1016/j.ejpain.2008.04.004

17. Mailis A, Wade J. Profile of Caucasian women with possible genetic predisposition to reflex sympathetic dystrophy: A pilot study. *Clin J Pain*. 1994;10(3):210–217. doi:10.1097/00002508-199409000-00007

18. Modarresi S, Aref-Eshghi E, Walton DM, MacDermid JC. Does a familial subtype of complex regional pain syndrome exist? Results of a systematic review. *Can J Pain*. 2019;3(1):157–166. doi:10.1080/24740527.2019.1637249

19. van de Beek WJ, Roep BO, van der Slik AR, Giphart MJ, van Hilten BJ. Susceptibility loci for complex regional pain syndrome. *Pain*. 2003;103(1–2):93–97. doi:10.1016/s0304-3959(02)00444-x

20. van Hilten JJ, van de Beek WJ, Roep BO. Multifocal or generalized tonic dystonia of complex regional pain syndrome: A distinct clinical entity associated with HLA-DR13. *Ann Neurol*. 2000;48(1):113–116. doi:10.1002/1531-8249(200007)48:1<113::aid-ana18>3.3.co;2-0

21. Kinoshita T, Abe RT, Hineno A, Tsunekawa K, Nakane S, Ikeda S. Peripheral sympathetic nerve dysfunction in adolescent Japanese girls following immunization with the human papillomavirus vaccine. *Intern Med*. 2015;53(19):2185–2200. doi:10.2169/internalmedicine.53.3133

22. Larson HJ, Wilson R, Hanley S, Parys A, Paterson P. Tracking the global spread of vaccine sentiments: The global response to Japan's suspension of its HPV vaccine recommendation. *Hum Vaccine Immunother*. 2014;10(9):2543–2550. doi:10.4161/21645515.2014.969618

23. Huygen F, Verschueren K, McCabe C, Stegmann JU, Zima J, Mahaux O, et al. Investigating reports of complex regional pain syndrome: An analysis of HPV-16/18-adjuvanted vaccine post-licensure data. *EBioMedicine*. 2015; 2(9):1114–1121. doi:10.1016/j.ebiom.2015.07.003

24. Weinbaum CM, Cano M. HPV vaccination and complex regional pain syndrome: Lack of evidence. *EBioMedicine*. 2015;2(9):1014–1015. doi:10.1016/j.ebiom.2015.08.030

25. Richards S, Chalkiadis G, Lakshman R, Buttery JP, Crawford NW. Complex regional pain syndrome following immunisation. *Arch Dis Child*. 2012;97(10):913–915. doi:10.1136/archdischild-2011-301307

26. Zhang J, Gungor S. Acute worsening of clinical presentation in CRPS after SARS-CoV-2 (COVID-19) vaccination: A case series. *Pain Manag*. 2022;12(3):249–254. doi:10.2217/pmt-2021-0089

27. McFarland AJ, Yousuf MS, Shiers S, Price TJ. Neurobiology of SARS-CoV-2 interactions with the peripheral nervous system: Implications for COVID-19 and pain. *Pain Rep*. 2021;6(1):e885. doi:10.1097/pr9.0000000000000885

2 How Do You Know the Cause?

Steven Mach and Salahadin Abdi

Case

A 50-year-old woman is concerned about her painful and swollen right leg. About 1 year ago, she fell off a ladder and sustained a fracture of her right ankle. She opted for nonsurgical management of her ankle fracture and was placed in a long-leg cast and on crutches for 2 months. After removal of her leg cast, she was advised to attend physical therapy, but she reports that she did not continue due to pain when moving her right leg. For the past 10 months, she has been mostly wheelchair-bound and needs assistance with standing and walking. She says that her leg was "never the same" after the cast came off and that it has been hot, swollen, and painful to gentle touch. On examination, the patient's right leg appears red (erythematous) and swollen (edematous), with a glossy shine up to her knee. Her foot and ankle have limited range of motion and are exquisitely tender to palpation.

What Do I Do Now?

DIAGNOSIS OF COMPLEX REGIONAL PAIN SYNDROME

This patient has a constellation of signs and symptoms characterized by unrelenting pain that appears out of proportion to the course of her injury (i.e., ankle fracture).[1] The pain extends beyond the region of her trauma, unconfined to a specific nerve or dermatome, and is associated with abnormal sensory, motor, sudomotor, vasomotor, and trophic changes. Without any other explanation for her symptoms, barring initial trauma as a cause, the patient's most likely diagnosis is complex regional pain syndrome (CRPS). Even so, other diagnoses may present with similar features and should also be explored.

The diagnosis of CRPS is made clinically on the basis of a history and physical examination. CRPS can be suspected when a patient presents with disproportionate pain and symptoms within 4–6 weeks of trauma. The patient here fulfills the Budapest Consensus Criteria for the clinical diagnosis of CRPS (sensitivity 82% and specificity 68%).[2] The criteria state that, for the diagnosis of CRPS, one must consider four categories: sensory, vasomotor, sudomotor/edema, and motor/trophic (see Table 2.1);[2,3] the patient must report one symptom in at least three of the four categories and display one sign in at least two of the four categories, with no other better clinical diagnosis. Pain is universally present in all cases. Two subtypes of CRPS exist: type I (i.e., reflex sympathetic dystrophy, the more common subtype) occurs without evidence of peripheral nerve injury, while type II (i.e., causalgia) occurs when nerve injury is present.

At this point, the history and physical examination suggest CRPS. Since CRPS is a clinical diagnosis, there is no gold standard lab test or technique to make the confirmation. Nonetheless, imaging modalities are available to help rule out other potential causes of pain. Plain radiographs (i.e., x-rays) can show patchy osteoporosis in CRPS. To get the most sensitive results, it is advised to image both analogous extremities (e.g., both hands or both feet) in the same x-ray to better detect any areas of osteoporosis in the affected limb (assuming the CRPS has not spread to the opposite side). After obtaining a single plain radiograph with the two feet side by side, you may note an increase in spotty bone loss in the patient's affected foot, though it is important to know that the sensitivity of this finding is very low.

In more sensitive imaging, bone scans (i.e., bone scintigraphy) can detect changes in bone and joints particularly due to infection, tumor, metabolic disease, metastatic disease, arthritis, and fractures. In patients with

TABLE 2.1 Budapest Consensus criteria for clinical diagnosis of CRPS

Symptom criteria	Symptoms (reported in history)
Patient must report at least **one symptom** in **three** of the four following **categories**	• **Sensory:** hyperesthesia and/or allodynia • **Vasomotor:** temperature asymmetry and/or skin color changes/asymmetry • **Sudomotor/Edema:** edema and/or sweating changes/asymmetry • **Motor/trophic:** decreased range of motion, and/or motor dysfunction (weakness, tremor, dystonia) and/or trophic changes (hair/skin/nail)
Sign criteria	Signs (observed on exam)
Patient must display at least **one sign** in **two** of the four following **categories**	• **Sensory:** hyperalgesia (to pinprick) and/or allodynia (to light touch, temperature, deep somatic pressure, or joint movement • **Vasomotor:** temperature asymmetry (>1 deg. C) or skin color changes/asymmetry • **Sudomotor/Edema:** edema and/or sweating changes/asymmetry • **Motor/trophic:** decreased range of motion, and/or motor dysfunction (weakness, tremor, dystonia) and/or trophic changes (hair/skin/nail)

Adapted with permission from Harden R. N., Oaklander A. L., Burton A. W., Perez R. S., Richardson K., Swan M., et al. (2013). Complex regional pain syndrome: practical diagnostic and treatment guidelines, 4th edition. *Pain Med.* 14(2):180–229. https://academic.oup.com/painmedicine/article/14/2/180/1824419.

CRPS who have active bone resorption, triple-phase bone scintigraphy can be a particularly useful tool to identify bony changes.[4] In the acute setting, a bone scan can be helpful if performed within the first 5 months after symptoms begin; CRPS patients can show increased uptake of radioactive tracer in joints distant to and unaffected by the initial trauma. In the case of our patient, a triple-phase bone scintigraphy shows patchy osteoporosis. It is important to remember that while bone scintigraphy can be useful, a normal scan does not rule out CRPS. Following results of the bone scan, the patient is started on a short-term bisphosphonate which provides her a small amount of pain relief.

Other advanced imaging modalities have limited usefulness. While CT scans can potentially show osteoporotic lesions, there is not much evidence proving its effectiveness in diagnosing CRPS. The diagnostic value of CT is limited given its risk-to-benefit ratio when weighing the financial cost and radiation dose to the patient. Similarly, while MRI can be helpful with ruling in other potential diagnoses, it is not useful in the setting of CRPS.

Our patient requests other tests to investigate the CRPS diagnosis. Given the common sudomotor and vasomotor changes of CRPS, autonomic tests such as the resting sweat output (RSO), resting skin temperature (RST), and quantitative sudomotor axon reflex test (QSART) have been used to evaluate patients suspected of having CRPS. While a small study demonstrated a 2° C temperature difference between the affected and unaffected limb, the serial measurements obtained every minute for several hours makes this clinical test impractical.

On a return visit, our patient says that she read on the internet about a "nerve block" that could help diagnose and treat her pain. Previous teaching dictated that temporary relief from a sympatholytic procedure, such as intravenous regional analgesia (i.e., Bier block) or a sympathetic nerve block (e.g., stellate ganglion or lumbar sympathetic nerve block) was required to diagnose CRPS. Currently, chemical sympatholysis is not part of the diagnostic criteria of CRPS because of the inconsistent role of the sympathetic nervous system in CRPS pathophysiology. While sympathetic mediated pain is possible, it is not always present in every patient.

After careful consideration, our patient decides to undergo a lumbar sympathetic nerve block. She experiences transient relief from her burning pain and hypersensitivity; however, within a few hours, hyperalgesia and allodynia return.

DIFFERENTIAL DIAGNOSIS OF COMPLEX REGIONAL PAIN SYNDROME

A month later, our patient returns. She says the treatment plan helps her pain a little, but she is wondering if any other diagnoses are possible. Given overlap of CRPS signs and symptoms with other disease states, a thorough assessment of a differential diagnosis is crucial in identifying and treating any reversible conditions. For example, painful peripheral neuropathy, such as diabetic peripheral neuropathy, can commonly present with pain, hypersensitivity, and trophic changes to the distal extremities. Another diagnosis to consider is infection of bone, joints, and soft tissue, which can appear similarly to CRPS. Patients with infections can present with pain, erythema, edema, and warmth. Common lab tests, such as erythrocyte sedimentation rate (ESR), C-reactive protein (CRP), and white blood cell (WBC) count, are often elevated with an infection. The patient decides to undergo lab tests for a complete blood count, ESR, and CRP, and the results return as normal.

Other potentially treatable conditions can mimic CRPS.[5] Acute compartment syndrome (ACS) is one such condition that is usually associated with substantial mechanical trauma of the long bones of the lower leg or forearm. ACS results from excessive pressure inside a fascial-bound compartment. A reduction in arterial blood flow causes tissue ischemia and necrosis of muscles and nerves. On exam, patients with ACS are expected to have pain out of proportion to the injury (especially with passive muscle stretch), tightness/swelling, and burning to the affected extremity. ACS is commonly a surgical emergency that warrants immediate decompression to alleviate the ischemia. Additionally, post-traumatic or post-surgical pain may appear in a distinct distribution of a peripheral nerve. The clearly demarcated distribution of pain should alert the provider to consider compromise of a specific nerve and usher prompt reevaluation by a surgical team and/or surgical exploration.

Patients with vascular disorders can also present similarly to CRPS. A patient who has chronic arterial insufficiency and hypoperfusion of the lower extremities may report cold feet with discoloration, cramping in the legs/feet, or pain that worsens with activity and improves with rest (i.e., vascular claudication). This suspicion is higher in patients with vascular disease risk factors such as smoking, increasing age, and atherosclerosis. Likewise, a vascular occlusion such as deep venous thrombosis (DVT) can also cause pain, swelling, and erythema, often in the lower extremities. A history of venous stasis, hypercoagulability, and physical examination showing tenderness to palpation, warmth, and redness is consistent with DVT. If found in conjunction with history and physical exam, a thrombus on Doppler ultrasonography would make DVT a more likely diagnosis than CRPS.

Another disorder to consider is thoracic outlet syndrome (TOC), which can result from compression of nerves (often brachial plexus) and/or blood vessels (often venous rather than arterial) of the upper extremity. It may present with swelling (usually without visible change), paresthesia, and erythema, commonly after overhead movement of the arms. For neurogenic TOC, a positive electrodiagnostic test has high specificity, although it is not as useful for screening purposes. Ultrasound, CT, and MRI can also help identify vascular compression, with x-ray being a useful initial test to show any bony cause of obstruction. Our patient is advised that these tests will likely return negative in CRPS, and she decides against further imaging.

Along the lines of vascular disorders, Reynaud's phenomenon (RP) can occur independently of or secondary to other autoimmune diseases. Much of the symptomatology of RP echoes that of CRPS. Triggers such as cold temperature and emotional stress can lead to an exaggerative vasoconstrictive response, as seen in RP. The syndrome is classically characterized by sharply demarcated skin changes on the fingers. RP is diagnosed if the fingers are abnormally sensitive to cold temperature and display color changes (to white and/or blue) when exposed to cold. Considering the similar presentation, the patient undergoes microvascular studies and autoimmune antibody testing for RP, and the results appear within normal ranges.

Another rare syndrome that can mimic CRPS is erythromelalgia, which is a clinical diagnosis based on signs and symptoms. Erythromelalgia is an acquired, though rarely inherited, disease that often affects adult women. It presents with transient episodes of red, hot, painful extremities that are triggered by heat or exercise and improve with cooling. It commonly affects the lower extremities (especially the feet) more than the upper extremities (often the hands), and rarely the face. Patients with erythromelalgia are predisposed to myeloproliferative disease, and even those without evidence of myeloproliferative disease at the time of diagnosis should be monitored for its development over time.

Rheumatologic issues can also present in the same way as CRPS. Diseases such as chronic rheumatoid arthritis (RA) affect the joint synovium. While the signs and symptoms of RA usually involve multiple joints (e.g., wrists, hands, shoulders, knees, and feet), CRPS is often limited to a single region or extremity. Furthermore, serology and highly specific laboratory markers (e.g., anti-citrullinated peptide) can help diagnose RA. Since our patient only has one affected limb, she is told that RA is less likely.

To identify further potential causes of this patient's symptoms, it is crucial to consider the behavioral-psycho-social component of pain. For example, pain, sensory derangements, and weakness are among the involuntary neurologic symptoms often reported in patients with conversion disorder; notably, their symptoms are not feigned, even in the absence of neurologic disease. On the other hand, a patient with factitious disorder can intentionally create physical findings or psychologic symptoms to assume the "sick role" or for secondary gain. When asked about her mood, the patient reports that she has been seeing a psychologist who has helped her to cope with the stressors of taking care of herself.

As you piece together our patient's history and exam, the discussion returns to establishing the best-fitting diagnosis for her unremitting right leg pain, redness, swelling, and immobility. Given the overlap of signs and symptoms of CRPS with other various diseases, ruling out further potential causes of pain, sensory, vasomotor, sudomotor, and motor dysfunction allows for management of any reversible conditions before arriving at the diagnosis of CRPS.

KEY POINTS TO REMEMBER

- Complex regional pain syndrome (CRPS) is a clinical diagnosis of exclusion.
- The Budapest Criteria for diagnosis of CRPS: the patient must report at least one symptom in three of four categories and display at least one sign in two of four categories (i.e., sensory, vasomotor, sudomotor/edema, and motor/trophic).
- Diagnostic testing is not required but could be helpful in identifying uncharacteristic cases or to exclude other diagnoses.
- The differential diagnosis for CRPS could include infection, erythromelalgia, compartment syndrome, peripheral vascular disease, deep vein thrombosis, vascular outlet syndrome, rheumatoid arthritis, Raynaud's phenomenon, conversion disorder, and factitious disorder, among others.

Suggested Reading

Abdi S. Complex regional pain syndrome in adults: Pathogenesis, clinical manifestations, and diagnosis. https://www.uptodate.com/contents/complex-regional-pain-syndrome-in-adults-pathogenesis-clinical-manifestations-and-diagnosis.

Harden RN, Oaklander AL, Burton AW, Perez RS, Richardson K, Swan M, et al. Complex regional pain syndrome: Practical diagnostic and treatment guidelines, 4th edition. *Pain Med*. 2013;14(2):180–229.

References

1. Abdi S. Complex regional pain syndrome in adults: Pathogenesis, clinical manifestations, and diagnosis. https://www.uptodate.com/contents/complex-regional-pain-syndrome-in-adults-pathogenesis-clinical-manifestations-and-diagnosis. Last updated September 3, 2024.
2. Harden RN, Bruehl S, Stanton-Hicks M, Wilson PR. Proposed new diagnostic criteria for complex regional pain syndrome. *Pain Med*. 2007;8(4):326–331.
3. Harden RN, Oaklander AL, Burton AW, Perez RS, Richardson K, Swan M, et al. Complex regional pain syndrome: Practical diagnostic and treatment guidelines, 4th edition. *Pain Med*. 2013;14(2):180–229.
4. Birklein F, O'Neill D, Schlereth T. Complex regional pain syndrome: An optimistic perspective. *Neurology*. 2015;84(1):89–96.
5. Turner-Stokes L, Goebel A. Complex regional pain syndrome in adults: Concise guidance. *Clin Med (Lond)*. 2011;11(6):596–600.

3 A Complex Disease

Steven Mach and Salahadin Abdi

Case

A 33-year-old woman presents to the pain clinic
with complaints of severe pain in her left arm, wrist,
and hand. Three years ago, she had surgical repair
of her fractured left distal radius and ulna after a
soccer injury. Since the injury, she has experienced
an intense burning and stabbing pain in her left hand
and arm. She also reports severe "electric shocks"
in her left arm from the rubbing of her clothing and
bedsheets on bare skin. The patient is distressed at
the appearance of her left arm and has noticed that
her hand appears mottled and blue and feels cold. In
addition, she reports stiffness and difficulty opening
and closing her left hand. On examination, the patient
exclaims in pain from light palpation of her left hand.
Her left arm is cool to the touch and is noticeably
glossy with increased hair growth compared to the
contralateral side. Furthermore, she has overgrown
fingernails. The patient wants to know more about the
reason for her symptoms.

What Do I Do Now?

PATHOPHYSIOLOGY OF COMPLEX REGIONAL PAIN SYNDROME

Uncovering the mechanisms underlying complex regional pain syndrome (CRPS) helps patients to understand links between pathology and clinical presentation. Our patient presents with numerous findings, both reported and observed on examination, that align with her existing diagnosis of CRPS (see Chapter 2, "How Do You Know the Cause?" for CRPS diagnosis and differential diagnosis). The pathogenesis of CRPS likely involves an array of factors (Table 3.1). A peripheral nerve injury is a distinguishing factor for CRPS type II and is absent in type I, yet pathophysiology is not a clear means of clinical distinction between the two subtypes.

One should first explore the role of inflammation in CRPS. Proinflammatory cytokines (such as interleukin [IL-]1β, IL-2, IL-6, and tumor necrosis factor [TNF]-α) and pronociceptive peptides (such as substance P, neuropeptide Y, and calcitonin gene-related peptide) appear to be involved in CRPS. Release of these inflammatory mediators and pain-producing peptides by peripheral nerves are a potential cause for the persistent pain, hyperalgesia (i.e., increased sensitivity to pain), and allodynia (i.e., pain from a normally painless stimulus) that classically describe CRPS. The aberrant firing of nerve impulses in the opposite direction from normal (e.g., from proximal to distal in sensory nociceptive neurons) causes the release of these inflammatory neuropeptides, a process known as *neurogenic inflammation*. Furthermore, abnormal communication between afferent and efferent neurons at the site of nerve injury has also been implicated in the formation of allodynia.

While inflammation can potentially cause CRPS pain, it might also explain the associated vasomotor signs and symptoms. It is proposed that the release of substance P from sensitized nerve fibers may trigger the release of vasoactive substances such as TNF-α and IL-1 from immune cells, which results in the arteriolar vasodilation and protein extravasation behind the erythema, edema, and temperature changes commonly seen in acute, "warm" CRPS. Modulation of the immune system has been a proposed therapeutic option by using biologics, such as anti-TNF antibodies and steroids to treat CRPS pain. After learning about these pharmacologic options, our patient decides against starting any additional medications.

TABLE 3.1 Pathophysiology of complex regional pain syndrome (CRPS)

Mechanism	Distinguishing features	Potential treatment options
Inflammation	• Proinflammatory cytokines (i.e., IL-1β, IL-2, IL-6, and TNF-α) elevated in the affected extremity and CSF • Decreased levels of anti-inflammatory cytokines (i.e., IL-10 and IL-4) in CRPS patients • Proinflammatory and nociceptive peptides (i.e., substance P, neuropeptide Y, and CGRP) mediate neurogenic inflammation • Communication between afferent and efferent nerves at site of injury can cause allodynia	• Improvement in symptoms with anti-TNF-α biologic therapy • Steroids (e.g., prednisone or prednisolone) for symptom management
Central sensitization	• Increased firing of somatosensory neuron in dorsal horn of spinal cord secondary to increased activity of nociceptive afferent nerves after injury • Sensitization of pain pathway via spinal cord leads to lower nociceptor activation threshold, hyperalgesia, and allodynia • Activation of glia in spinal cord leads to persistent nociception	Changes seen in somatosensory cortex in fMRI reversible with symptom treatment
Sympathetic nervous system	• Autonomic dysregulation related to catecholamine hypersensitivity • Expression of adrenergic receptors on nociceptive fibers after tissue/nerve injury • Increased sensitivity of pain producing receptors to epinephrine • Activation of SNS modulated by cortical brain centers can result in pain and changes to vasomotor tone	Pain sensation and sensitivity to catecholamines can be blocked by sympatholytic agents
Genetic factors	• Increased frequency of *HLA-DQ1* in patients with CRPS type I • Increased frequency of *HLA-DR13* in patients with CRPS that progressed to multifocal or generalized dystonia	Potential for HLA genotyping to detect risk factors
Autoimmune	Higher rates of ANA and IG autoantibodies against autonomic neurons in CRPS patients	IVIG for treatment of pain

ANA, antinuclear antibodies; CGRP, calcitonin gene-related peptide; fMRI, functional magnetic resonance imaging; HLA, human leukocyte antigen; IG, immunoglobulin G; IVIG, intravenous immunoglobulin; SNS, sympathetic nervous system; TNF, tumor necrosis factor.

Exploring the multiple mechanisms underlying CRPS uncovers the possible role of central nervous system (CNS) sensitization in causing pain and allodynia. Persistent or noxious stimuli, tissue damage, or nerve injury causes increased firing of pain-sensing afferent nerves, which, in turn, leads to increased activation of somatosensory neurons in the dorsal horn of the spinal cord. Local mediators of central sensitization include nociceptive peptides such as substance P (acting on G protein-coupled receptors) and neurotransmitters such as glutamate (acting on N-methyl-D-aspartate receptors). Increased pain signaling from the spinal cord to the brain may lead to prolonged or exaggerated responses to pain (i.e., hyperalgesia) as well as activation of pain receptors in response to normally painless or low-intensity stimuli (i.e., allodynia). Following sensitization, pain-sensing fibers develop a lower activation threshold to peripheral stimuli and can even fire in the absence of painful or noxious inputs. Moreover, glia in the spinal cord can also become activated. These glial cells (such as the microglia and astrocytes that maintain structural integrity and homeostasis of neurons) have an upregulation of surface receptors to the pronociceptive cytokines and peptides responsible for the induction and maintenance of persistent pain.

As more is understood about central sensitization, techniques have been applied to detect these changes. In fact, the structural adaptations in the CNS have been reflected on advanced imaging, such as functional (fMRI); patients with CRPS can show reversible changes in the primary somatosensory cortex (S1) contralateral to the affected extremity. These cortical changes may result from connections between adjacent neurons. The communication of neighboring nerves in the somatosensory cortex might provide an explanation for the "regional" distribution of CRPS, which often affects the general area of an extremity rather than a distinct nerve distribution.

The role of the autonomic nervous system in CRPS remains indeterminate. While classic teaching attributes the common sympathetic features of CRPS to excessive sympathetic outflow, current understanding suggests that peripheral pain receptors display hypersensitivity to catecholamines. After an inciting event or tissue trauma, expression of adrenergic receptors on afferent nociceptive fibers results in a coupling of the sympathetic nervous system (SNS) to pain-producing pathways. Neurons innervating injured tissue can show an exaggerated pain response to epinephrine and other substances released by local sympathetic nerves. In effect, SNS activity can trigger nociceptive firing. Increased sensitivity to catecholamines has been associated with increased rates of spontaneous pain and hyperalgesia in patients with CRPS.

The feedback loop between the SNS and cortical centers can also result in peripheral vascular changes. Initial sympathetic hyperstimulation may cause subsequent sympathetic malfunction that results in impaired vasomotor tone. This is a possible explanation for the warm, red extremity seen in acute CRPS. Paradoxically, in chronic CRPS, increased vasoconstriction has been observed even with decreased levels of catecholamines. The subsequent upregulation of peripheral adrenoreceptors on vascular smooth muscle causes an exaggerated response to the low/normal levels of circulating catecholamines that may be present. In addition to adrenergic hypersensitivity and endothelial dysfunction, decreased levels of vasodilating agents (such as nitric oxide) have been implicated in the development of the characteristic cold, blue limb of chronic CRPS. The increased adrenergic sensitivity is the basis for improvement in pain following a sympathetic nerve block. After discussing the potential risks and benefits of a sympatholytic procedure, our case study patient decides to undergo a stellate ganglion block, which provides temporary pain relief and improves the range of motion in her arm.

She begins to wonder if she could have inherited CRPS or if her family is at risk for developing similar symptoms. The pathogenesis of CRPS may involve genetic factors encoding immune function. Serologic human leukocyte antigen (HLA) typing for class I and II major histocompatibility (MHC) antigens has shown an association between CRPS type I and an increased frequency of *HLA-DQ1* (a gene that involves the repair of damaged neural tissue). In addition, CRPS patients who developed multifocal or generalized tonic dystonia had higher frequencies of the *HLA-DR13* allele. It remains unclear whether the predisposition for CRPS is related to the genetic loci themselves or is linked to nearby genes. Furthermore, it is uncertain if the HLA alleles play a role in developing CRPS or the onset and maintenance of disease. With no clear association between HLA typing and phenotypic symptoms, the patient decides to defer genetic testing.

Research into other avenues for treatment reveals that CRPS has a possible autoimmune component. Compared to the general population, patients with CRPS have a higher prevalence of antinuclear antibodies (ANA). Nonetheless, the link between the presence of ANA and signs/symptoms remains unknown. Other studies have demonstrated the role of autoantibodies. Immunoglobulin-G (Ig-G) from CRPS patients had increased rates of binding to adrenoreceptors on sympathetic cells compared to healthy controls. Sensitization of peripheral nociceptors secondary to Ig-G autoantibodies to adrenoreceptors may explain the induction and maintenance of pain and hyperalgesia. This is one possible rationale for the role of therapeutic intravenous immunoglobulin (IVIG) for CRPS pain relief. However, outcomes have been disappointing so far.

Our patient is told that the multiple mechanisms underlying the pathophysiology of CRPS are most likely intertwined. Connections between inflammation, peripheral and central sensitization, autonomic dysfunction, catecholamine hypersensitivity, genetic factors, and autoimmune regulation all offer possible explanations for the cause of CRPS. The effect of each factor on each individual patient likely differs on a case-by case basis. A better understanding of the pathogenesis of CRPS will aid in correlating mechanisms to risk factors, clinical presentation, diagnostic tools, and treatment options.

KEY POINTS TO REMEMBER

- The pathophysiology of complex regional pain syndrome (CRPS) is unclear but likely involves both peripheral and central nervous system mechanisms, including dysfunctional pain perception.
- Increased transmission in the dorsal horn of the spinal cord and cortical sensory and motor changes (cortical reorganization) may lead to a persistent pain condition.
- Coupling of autonomic and nociceptive somatic nerves can result in persistent pain.
- Genetic factors and autoimmune antibodies to autonomic neurons play a role in CRPS.

Suggested Reading

Bruehl S. An update on the pathophysiology of complex regional pain syndrome. *Anesthesiology*. 2010;113(3):713–725.

Bussa M, Guttilla D, Lucia M, Mascaro A, Rinaldi S. Complex regional pain syndrome type I: A comprehensive review. *Acta Anaesthesiol Scand*. 2015;59(6):685–697.

Jänig W, Baron R. Complex regional pain syndrome: Mystery explained? *Lancet Neurol*. 2003;2(11):687–697.

Marinus J, Moseley GL, Birklein F, Baron R, Maihöfner C, Kingery WS, et al. Clinical features and pathophysiology of complex regional pain syndrome. *Lancet Neurol*. 2011;10(7):637–648.

4 The Standard Approach

Sajan Shah, Allie Van Nuys,
Brittney Jones, Corinne Cooley,
Emily Moore, and Michael Leong

Case

A 34-year-old woman presents to the clinic for chronic right foot pain. She had a right ankle sprain 4 years ago managed with immobilization in a cast. Despite initial conservative management, her pain continued to worsen. She described her pain back then as right foot burning pain with significant swelling, redness, skin mottling, and coolness to touch. She also reported sensitivity to light touch, difficulty wearing socks and shoes, weakness, and tremor at the time. Her pain was initially treated by a combination of desensitization, orthopedic physical therapy, regular lumbar sympathetic blocks, and medications that include duloxetine and tramadol. She also underwent a few rounds of lidocaine systemic infusion. She is concerned that her current regimen is no longer helping the pain in her foot. She was able to walk without assistance but now sometimes requires a cane.

What Do I Do Now?

DIAGNOSIS

This case represents a typical presentation of complex regional pain syndrome (CRPS). Providers often implement the Budapest Criteria to support the diagnosis of CRPS.[1] Continuing pain disproportionate to the inciting event, as described by the patient, is one of the supporting features. Additionally, the patient demonstrates allodynia, differences in skin temperature and color, swelling, and tremor. These signs and symptoms fulfill the second part of the Budapest criteria. Finally, the last component of the criteria, which often complicates the diagnosis, is the requirement that no other diagnosis can better explain the signs and symptoms.[1] Providers will generally complete a comprehensive workup in the form of additional labs, imaging, and physical examination to rule out obvious musculoskeletal injuries, rheumatological conditions, and other conditions explaining the patient's presentation.

In this case, further workup of the patient yielded negative results, and the diagnosis of CRPS was confirmed. Initial management of this patient involved conventional therapy, which is a multimodal approach of physical and occupational therapy, medical drug therapy, and psychiatric therapy. While eliminating pain and discomfort is the ideal goal, in practice, this is not often achievable. A realistic goal is to make the symptoms tolerable enough to enable the patient to participate in physical therapy, eventually facilitating a return to normal function in the affected limb.

PHYSICAL AND OCCUPATIONAL THERAPY

In the acute phase of CRPS, physical and occupational therapy are often first-line treatments.[2] CRPS is a painful condition that has a high impact on a person's quality of life and can lead to high levels of disability.[3] Whether the CRPS is in the upper or lower extremity, it can affect the ability to use the limb for gait, grasping/reaching, and daily activities, as well as for social participation, recreational activities, work, and sports. Longitudinal studies have found that strength and proprioceptive impairments that alter gait can be sustained for years after CRPS presents in the lower extremity.[4] It is essential to have rehabilitation professionals as part of the patient's healthcare team as soon as possible, taking into consideration the individual's functional goals and addressing physical impairments.

Interventions by a physical therapist that have been studied include:

- Cortically directed sensory-motor rehabilitation strategies (e.g., graded motor imagery [GMI], mirror therapy, sensory-motor retuning, tactile discrimination training, and sensorimotor discrimination)[5–8]
- Manual therapy (e.g., mobilization, manipulation, massage, desensitization)[9]
- Therapeutic exercise and progressive loading regimens (including hydrotherapy)
- Electrotherapy (e.g., transcutaneous electrical nerve stimulation [TENS])
- Therapeutic ultrasound, interferential, shortwave diathermy, laser
- Physiotherapist-administered education (e.g., pain neuroscience education). Pain neuroscience education helps patients better understand the biological processes underlying their pain in a way that positively changes pain perceptions and attitudes for rehabilitation processes.[9]
- Graded exposure therapy (GEXP), in which the clinician works collaboratively with the patient to help the patient make a cognitive shift from "protection" of the painful limb to "exposure" or "use" of the painful limb for treatment to be successful; dropout for this type of therapy is high[10]
- Virtual reality: Several pilot studies have been published evaluating the feasibility of using virtual reality for short-term improvements in pain after virtual reality interventions, but provide limited data on objective or long-term changes for CRPS[11,12]

Treatment approaches that the rehabilitation professional might use for a person with CRPS have different degrees of efficacy. A 2022 systematic review of 34 randomized controlled trials (RCTs) with 1,339 participants evaluated a variety of physical therapy interventions for CRPS to improve pain and disability/function over time.[2] Unfortunately, a high risk of bias (27/34 trials) led to research evidence of very low quality due to study limitations and imprecision. Only 20 case reports of CRPS have been reported among athletes in the literature, with a higher prevalence in females than males (15:5).[13] Of the rehabilitation interventions, GMI and mirror therapy were most promising, with statistically significant improvements in pain and disability. Smaller studies have found GEXP superior to conventional rehabilitation for CRPS to improve disability in patients with high pain-related fear.[14]

Occupational therapists also play an important role on comprehensive pain management teams with a specific focus on patient function.[15] Through engagement in health-promoting daily routines, occupational therapists seek to address underlying disability, functional impairments, and pain in patients living with a diagnosis of CRPS.[16]

Occupational therapists are skilled in assessing multiple domains of functioning and taking into consideration client, environmental, and occupational factors. The occupational therapy evaluation assesses current level of performance in activities of daily living (ADLs), instrumental activities of daily living (IADLs), functional mobility, sleep, sexual function, leisure engagement, work performance, and social participation. Many factors contribute to clients' abilities to engage in these daily routines, and objective measurements of physical functioning, including range of motion, sensation, edema/lymphedema, skin changes, and strength, are considered as building blocks for engagement. Occupational therapists consider how the physical environment—including access to adaptive equipment and available social support—either facilitates or further inhibits functioning. The evaluation process often includes objective tests and measurements such as:

- The Canadian Occupational Performance Measure (COPM) and the Fear Avoidance Hierarchy to elicit functional goal setting[17,18]
- The Role Checklist Version 3 to assess psychosocial functioning, participation, and satisfaction in valued roles[19]
- The Adolescent/Adult Sensory Profile to establish a holistic view of sensory processing as well as specific sites for future intervention [8,20,21]

Immediately after the case patient's diagnosis of CRPS was confirmed, physical and occupational therapy were each scheduled once weekly for 4 weeks. The physical and occupational therapists collaborated with the patient to develop a plan aimed at addressing the areas of impairment identified in an evaluation. Evidence-based interventions included patient and family education targeting pain neuroscience, self-management strategies, activity pacing, environmental and task modifications, and caregiver training with trusted family and friends.[9,22,23] The occupational therapist facilitated ADL and IADL retraining with an emphasis on a return to valued leisure activities, social participation, and important roles identified through the COPM and the Role Checklist Version 3.[17,18] The physical therapist led manual therapy, therapeutic exercise, progressive loading regimens, and GMI. In partnership with the physical therapist, the occupational therapist worked with the patient to establish a home activity program that carried over GMI exercises and sensory discrimination/desensitization principles to facilitate somatosensory cortical reorganization.[6–8,21,24–27] As the patient's symptoms began to improve, the occupational therapist facilitated graded activity and task exposure utilizing information from the Fear Avoidance Hierarchy.[28] With time, sessions were reduced to biweekly, giving the patient increased time to practice the integration of various self-management strategies into her daily activities with greater focus in occupational therapy on collaborative problem-solving through challenges and progressing in her home activity program.

The patient became nonadherent to her therapy regimen over time. She developed worsening symptoms with reduced effectiveness of her ongoing therapy, and she required walking assistance, which led to her most recent presentation to the clinic. The importance of physical and occupational therapy was reinforced, and she was referred again to these specialists.

PHARMACOLOGICAL/MEDICAL THERAPY

Pharmacotherapy is essential in the management of a patient with CRPS. The key focus with pharmaceuticals is to relieve pain and improve function. Medications also play a critical role in facilitating a patient's ability to participate in physical therapy. In this patient, as symptoms worsened, she was not able to participate in physical therapy effectively. This led to the addition of pharmaceutical therapy. Pharmacological management of CRPS is complex, and no universally applicable approach is available due to tremendous interpatient variability in presentation and response to treatment. Augmenting this complexity is the lack of high-quality RCTs in the management of CRPS. Nonetheless, initial pharmacological therapy is focused on targeting neuropathic pain and inflammation.

For patients presenting with a neuropathic pain component of their CRPS symptoms, anticonvulsants such as gabapentin or pregabalin are often initiated. Surprisingly, there is no evidence to support the use of these medications. One RCT randomized 58 patients to either two 3-week treatment periods with gabapentin and placebo separated by a 2-week washout period.[29] The results of this study demonstrated that gabapentin produced a mild reduction in pain initially, but eventually the beneficial effect waned. Patients with sensory deficits at baseline did report reduction in the sensory deficit with gabapentin use. A separate systematic review published in 2021 listed three studies that found an improvement in pain; however, the evidence was not sufficient to recommend use for every patient with CRPS.[30] These small benefits are outweighed by the risks of the medication. In fact, respiratory dysfunction is a major concern with the use of gabapentin, and the US Food and Drug Administration (FDA) has published a warning regarding this side effect.[31] The use of anticonvulsant medications in treating CRPS appears to be limited to a subset of patients who have a neuropathic component to their pain and a sensory deficit; close monitoring for side effects is essential.

Tricyclic antidepressants (TCAs) and serotonin and noradrenaline reuptake inhibitors (SNRIs) may also target the neuropathic component of CRPS pain; however, there are no studies at this time investigating their use specifically in CRPS. The benefit of these antidepressants is demonstrated in neuropathic pain conditions in numerous studies.[32] Additionally, pain is often augmented by underlying depression, which developed in our case patient. Using medications such as amitriptyline and duloxetine results in a dual mechanism of action toward pain and mood, resulting in a synergistic improvement in overall pain in patients.[32] Although studies showing the efficacy of TCAs and SNRIs in CRPS are pending, they are a reasonable adjunct to a multimodal approach to the management of CRPS symptoms barring development of side effects.

Previous biopsy studies have demonstrated that tissue inflammation is a component of the pathophysiology of CRPS, thus prompting the use of anti-inflammatory agents.[33] Anti-inflammatory therapy consists of glucocorticoids, nonsteroidal anti-inflammatory drugs (NSAIDs), bisphosphonates, and free radical scavengers.

Overall, evidence for the use of glucocorticoids is minimal and favors a short course of an oral glucocorticoid medication in the early stages of CRPS.[33,34] Previous trials comparing oral glucocorticoids to placebo demonstrated a beneficial effect of the medication in outcomes such as pain, edema, and function.[35,36] While these trials were small in size and had significant methodological limitations, they did show benefit of oral glucocorticoid therapy. Additionally, a previous RCT by Kalita, Vajpayee, and Misra[37] showed that oral glucocorticoids are more effective in improving CRPS symptoms than are NSAIDs. In a patient who appears to have an inflammatory component to their CRPS, a short course of oral glucocorticoids in the acute phase of CRPS is recommended. There is a lack of evidence for the long-term use of oral corticosteroids in the management of chronic CRPS, and it is reasonable to assume that the risk outweighs the benefit given the side-effect profile of glucocorticoids.

NSAIDs are thought to be effective in the management of CRPS via the inhibition of COX and subsequent decreased synthesis of prostaglandins attenuating nociception.[38] There is a dearth of studies on the use of NSAIDs in CRPS, and the existing studies are not robust. One small RCT by Breuer et al.[38] comparing parecoxib to placebo in the treatment of CRPS showed no significant benefit of parecoxib in the improvement of CRPS pain, casting doubt on the role of COX-2 on the manifestation of CRPS. As mentioned earlier, NSAIDs were shown to be inferior to glucocorticoids in CRPS.[37] The lack of benefit of NSAIDs is only demonstrated in small trials, which is likely why expert guidelines draw on previous clinical experience to continue to recommend the addition of NSAIDs to multimodal therapy of CRPS.[39]

Free radical scavengers are another drug type within the category of anti-inflammatory medications for the treatment of CRPS. Inflammation can theoretically lead to the production of free radicals contributing to the tissue destruction seen in CRPS. Conflicting evidence exists for the use of free radical scavengers: 50% dimethyl sulfoxide (DMSO) has been previously studied in the form of a fatty cream applied for 2 months in patients with CRPS.[40] In this study, reflex sympathetic dystrophy scores were significantly better in the DMSO group compared to placebo.[40] Similarly, in another study, a 3-week course of DMSO 50% also showed significant improvement in pain, disability, and function compared to intravenous regional blockade with ismelin.[41] Both these studies are outdated and small in sample sizes. A more recent RCT compared DMSO to N-acetylcysteine (NAC) and placebo.[42] Both treatment arms of the study demonstrated significant improvement in Injury Severity Scores compared to placebo, and there was no statistically significant difference in Injury Severity Scores between DMSO and NAC. Strong evidence to support the use of free radical scavengers in the management of CRPS is lacking, and the treatment would not be suggested for the management of this patient.

One of the most well-studied and evidence-supported therapeutic options in CRPS is a bisphosphonate medication. From the perspective of pain, bisphosphonates were traditionally used to treat pain in bone diseases through their anti-osteoclastic properties. Due to the bone demineralization present in CRPS, initially there was consideration that bisphosphonates may improve pain and function in CRPS via inhibition of bone loss. More recently, bisphosphonates have been thought to have a greater anti-inflammatory role in the treatment of CRPS via decreased production of proinflammatory mediators.[43,44] Supporting evidence for bisphosphonate therapy in CRPS treatment comes in the form of several small RCTs. A 3-day intravenous infusion of alendronate showed improved pain, swelling, edema, and function compared to placebo.[45] Daily oral alendronate also demonstrated improved pain, pressure tolerance, and mobility compared to placebo.[46] Ten-day infusions of both intravenous neridronate and clodronate demonstrated improved pain and reduced allodynia and hyperalgesia.[47,48] Interestingly, a single dose of intravenous pamidronate also improved pain scores compared to placebo.[49] Bisphosphonate therapy was compared to oral glucocorticoid treatment as well and demonstrated similar efficacy in improving pain scores, which is beneficial considering the safer side-effect profile of bisphosphonates compared to glucocorticoids.[50] It is also important to note that not all of these studies selected for individuals with evidence of bone demineralization. Therefore, despite the evidence lacking larger sample sizes and longer duration of follow-up, current evidence supports the use of bisphosphonates in treating CRPS, and the treatment would be recommended in the case patient.

Adjuvant topical therapies are not well-studied in CRPS patients. However, given the overall low side-effect profile of these topical agents, they are often used first-line to assist in reducing CRPS-associated pain. These therapies include topical lidocaine, capsaicin cream, and topical NSAIDs. These agents have a few studies supporting their individual use, but the data are not robust, thus the evidence is weak.[40] Some providers compound special formulations with a combination of the aforementioned topical agents along with even ketamine powder; however, there is no evidence to support ketamine's use.

Opioids are generally avoided but are added to the treatment regimen if existing therapy does not provide analgesia sufficient to enable the patient to participate in physical therapy. The use of opioids in chronic noncancer pain in general is controversial.[40] When they are prescribed, concerns arise regarding tolerance, opioid use disorder, and overdose. Some experts also suggest that long-term, high-dose opioid use could lead to hyperalgesia or worsen allodynia.[51] For this reason, any clinician prescribing opioids to patients with CRPS should establish a strong therapeutic relationship with their patients and set patient expectations and treatment goals.[52] Additionally, opioid dose escalations are not recommended, especially as there is currently insufficient evidence for the use of opioids in the treatment of CRPS-related pain.[40]

For our case patient, it appears that tramadol and duloxetine had controlled her pain at first. Over time, though, her symptoms worsened. She again was not able to effectively participate in physical therapy, and further titration of her medications was necessary. Her provider discussed at length the natural course of CRPS and emphasized that chronic use of opioids for management of nonmalignant chronic pain is best avoided. A plan was set to first optimize pain control with adjunctive medications and then wean off opioids over time. This patient was also unsure whether her duloxetine was helping her pain, and this medication was weaned off her regimen. A TCA and alendronate were the next options to be considered.

PAIN PSYCHOLOGY

Pain psychology is an essential component of a multimodal approach toward pain. Our patient was not referred to pain psychology at initial diagnosis;

however, when she returned with worsening function and pain at her most recent visit to the clinic, she was then referred to pain psychology.

For centuries, pain was conceptualized as a primarily sensory phenomenon, stemming from nociceptive or neuropathic origins. This one-sided conceptualization of pain, illustrated by Descartes in *The Treatise on Man* in 1662,[53] prevailed as the predominant doctrine governing pain theories and practices. While nociception may lead to pain, remarkably, pain can occur without nociception or sensory input.[54] To reflect the multifactorial genesis of pain, the International Association for the Study of Pain (IASP) defines pain as, "An unpleasant sensory and emotional experience associated with, or resembling that associated with, actual or potential tissue damage."[55] The IASP's updated pain definition highlights the complex interplay of neurobiological, psychological, environmental, and cognitive factors that modulate and influence pain perception. Nuanced explanations of pain also align with complex pain syndromes, such as CRPS, that transcend purely nociceptive or neuropathic underpinnings.

Beyond nociceptive and neuropathic pain lies *nociplastic pain*, a pathophysiologically-based term to more accurately describe and validate the experience of patients with significant pain and altered nociceptive function despite no apparent nociceptor activation or neuropathy.[56] CRPS is considered the only neuropathic and nociplastic condition.[57] At the crux of nociplastic pain is the concept of *plasticity*, or alterations that occur when the nervous system reorganizes itself, changing its structure and function.[58] Consequently, the nervous system can "learn" chronic pain.

Applying neuroplasticity to CRPS, research demonstrates that changes in brain representation shift from nociceptive to emotional circuits, emphasizing alterations in sensory and motor maps and maladaptive cortical plasticity.[59] The plasticity of the nervous system was postulated in the *gate control theory*, which provides a physiological explanation for processing pain information and factors that modulate sensory input by the "spinal gate" mechanism.[60] Innovatively, Melzack and Wall[60] considered the role of psychopathology in the opening of the "pain gate," including "past experience, attention, and emotion influenced pain response and perception by acting on the gate control system."

Given the complex interplay of emotional factors in the pain experience, it is imperative for providers to assess factors that contribute to negative mental states, decreased functioning, and pain intensity. For example, pain sensitization involves Pavlovian conditioning or associative learning, leading to changes in pain sensitivity, pain tolerance, and pain threshold.[61] With repeated noxious stimuli, associative learning, and sensitization, pain often becomes a feared stimulus, leading to fear conditioning. Patients with CRPS often demonstrate pain catastrophizing, an exaggerative and negative mental representation of pain with a tendency to focus on pain with the perception that pain is unmanageable.[62,63] Fear conditioning and related pain beliefs (e.g., pain catastrophizing) prevail in pain-related disability, with fear-avoidance experienced in regard to activities and elicited fear in anticipation of pain.[64] With pain serving as a feared stimulus and subsequent response to feared stimuli, an iterative process of avoidance, fear, and pain spirals into inactivity and disability. With the synergistic and complex mechanisms involved in the development and maintenance of chronic pain, particularly nociplastic pain, an integrated, biopsychosocial approach to pain management is paramount to effectively address CRPS.

A number of mental health conditions can co-occur with CRPS, including depression, anxiety, post-traumatic stress disorder (PTSD), and somatic symptom disorder. The consideration of psychiatric comorbidities when treating individuals experiencing CRPS is critical due to the potentially exacerbating and interfering impact of mood dysfunction, anxiety, and post-traumatic symptoms. Depression is the most common psychiatric illness to present with chronic pain more broadly and has also been noted to specifically occur in patients experiencing CRPS, such as in our case patient.[65,66] Identification and treatment of depressive symptoms are important because symptoms can reduce pain tolerance and interfere with multidisciplinary treatment adherence. In addition, research has demonstrated that depressed mood both predicts pain and results from pain, highlighting the complex relationship between these two factors.[67] The prevalence of anxiety disorders within the chronic pain population is significantly elevated.[68] There is a paucity of data specifically examining comorbidity between CRPS and anxiety; however, patients with CRPS often experience pain-related anxiety which prompts activity avoidance and often, in turn, exacerbates pain. With regard to PTSD, one study has reported a higher prevalence in CRPS patients, but more data are needed to support this conclusion.[69]

Behavioral health interventions are a critical aspect of effective multidisciplinary care. They have demonstrated value in addressing comorbid psychological symptoms associated with CRPS, increasing functioning, and reducing pain. Behavioral health interventions utilize a biopsychosocial framework, which is particularly useful in understanding and treating the psychological symptoms often experienced by CRPS patients. Treatment can be offered in an individual or group format either in-person or through online delivery to increase access. Although limited research has investigated the behavioral health needs of CRPS patients, there is solid evidence for a number of psychological approaches in the treatment of chronic pain. Overall, behavioral health interventions foster motivation, support treatment adherence, target problematic cognitions, and promote active coping. Cognitive-behavioral therapy (CBT) is a highly regarded intervention and the most commonly implemented psychological treatment for chronic pain.[70] CBT directly addresses thoughts, emotions, and behaviors related to the pain experience. The main components of CBT for chronic pain are psychoeducation, pain neuroscience education, relaxation training, cognitive restructuring, sleep hygiene, behavioral activation, and activity pacing. Acceptance and commitment therapy (ACT), a third-wave CBT approach, has also demonstrated efficacy in chronic pain populations.[71] ACT is a therapeutic approach that aims to foster acceptance of suffering and promotes engagement in a rich and meaningful life despite the presence of pain. ACT does not seek to control or cure pain, which juxtaposes it against CBT, which aims to regulate pain experience. The core components of ACT are acceptance, contact with the present moment, values, cognitive defusion, committed action, and self-as-context. This approach has been suggested to be especially beneficial in CRPS due to the severity of symptoms and associated functional limitations.[72,73]

Our patient was started on CBT by the pain psychologist to whom she was referred as a part of her multimodal therapy. The patient noted significant improvement in her ability to cope with her pain and improvement in her relationships as well.

SUMMARY

After this patient's return to the clinic for worsening pain and need for ambulation assistance, the following changes were enacted: she was re-referred to and encouraged to participate in physical and occupational therapy, and she was weaned off tramadol and duloxetine; nortriptyline was initiated, and she underwent CBT with the pain clinic. This treatment strategy has been successful in restoring her full function: she is back at work as a laboratory technician, goes on regular hikes, and occasionally goes jogging. She was even able to run a 5K race.

KEY POINTS TO REMEMBER

- *Consider multimodal therapy.* A combination of physical therapy, medication management, and behavioral health interventions can have a more effective impact on a patient's improvement compared to any one method alone.
- *Tailor treatment plans to individual patients.* Complex regional pain syndrome (CRPS) is a complex condition with a variety of symptoms and comorbidities. Treatment plans should be tailored to the individual patient, taking into account their specific symptoms, medical history, and psychological profile. Pain management specialists should work closely with patients to develop personalized treatment plans that address their unique needs.
- *Monitor medication use.* The use of opioids and other pain medications for CRPS should be carefully monitored, especially in patients with comorbid conditions or a history of substance abuse. Patients should be weaned off opioids if possible, and other medications such as tricyclic antidepressants or anticonvulsants may be more appropriate.
- *Consider comorbid psychological symptoms.* Patients with CRPS often experience comorbid psychological symptoms such as anxiety and depression. These symptoms should be addressed in treatment plans, and behavioral health interventions such as cognitive-behavioral therapy or acceptance and commitment therapy may be effective.
- *Address functional limitations.* Patients with CRPS often experience functional limitations that can impact their daily

lives. Physical therapy and occupational therapy can be effective in improving mobility and functionality. Pain management specialists should work with these therapists to develop comprehensive treatment plans.

- *Educate patients about pain.* Patients should be educated about the biology of pain and how it relates to their symptoms. This can help them better understand their condition and improve their coping strategies.

Suggested Reading

Duong S, Bravo D, Todd KJ, Finlayson RJ, Tran Q. Treatment of complex regional pain syndrome: An updated systematic review and narrative synthesis. *Can J Anesth/ J canadien danesthésie.* 2018;65(6):658–684.

Hudson J, Lake E, Spruit E, Terrell M, Cooper K, McFawn C, et al. Comprehensive rehabilitation of patients with complex regional pain syndrome. *Complex Regional Pain Syndrome.* 2021. https://doi.org/10.1007/978-3-030-75373-3_7

Smart KM, Wand BM, O'Connell NE. Physiotherapy for pain and disability in adults with complex regional pain syndrome (CRPS) types I and II. *Cochrane Database Syst Rev.* 2016;2:CD010853. https://doi.org/10.1002/14651858.CD010853.pub2

Taylor SS, Noor N, Urits I, Paladini A, Sadhu MS, Gibb C, et al. Complex regional pain syndrome: A comprehensive review. *Pain Ther.* 2021;10(2):875–892.

References

1. Goebel A, Bisla J, Carganillo R, Cole C, Frank B, Gupta R, et al. Research diagnostic criteria (the Budapest Criteria) for complex regional pain syndrome, A randomised placebo-controlled Phase III multicentre trial: Low-dose intravenous immunoglobulin treatment for long-standing complex regional pain syndrome (LIPS trial). *NIHR Journals Library.* 2017. https://www.ncbi.nlm.nih.gov/books/NBK464482/

2. Smart KM, Wand BM, O'Connell NE. Physiotherapy for pain and disability in adults with complex regional pain syndrome (CRPS) types I and II. *Cochrane Database Syst Rev.* 2016;2:CD010853. https://doi.org/10.1002/14651858.CD010853.pub2

3. Taylor SS, Noor N, Urits I, Paladini A, Sadhu MS, Gibb C, et al. Complex regional pain syndrome: A comprehensive review. *Pain Ther.* 2021;10(2):875–892. https://doi.org/10.1007/s40122-021-00279-4

4. Mouraux D, Lenoir C, Tuna T, Brassinne E, Sobczak S. The long-term effect of complex regional pain syndrome type 1 on disability and quality of life after foot injury. *Disability Rehabil.* 2021;43(7):967–975. https://doi.org/10.1080/09638 288.2019.1650295

5. Moseley GL. Graded motor imagery is effective for long-standing complex regional pain syndrome: A randomised controlled trial. *Pain.* 2004;108(1–2):192–198. https://doi.org/10.1016/j.pain.2004.01.006

6. Méndez-Rebolledo G, Gatica-Rojas V, Torres-Cueco R, Albornoz-Verdugo M, Guzmán-Muñoz E. Update on the effects of graded motor imagery and mirror therapy on complex regional pain syndrome type 1: A systematic review. *J Back Musculoskel Rehabil.* 2017;30(3):441–449. https://doi.org/10.3233/BMR-150500

7. Quintal I, Poiré-Hamel L, Bourbonnais D, Dyer JO. Management of long-term complex regional pain syndrome with allodynia: A case report. *J Hand Ther.* 2018;31(2):255–264. https://doi.org/10.1016/j.jht.2018.01.012

8. Quintal I, Carrier A, Packham T, Bourbonnais D, Dyer JO. Tactile stimulation programs in patients with hand dysesthesia after a peripheral nerve injury: A systematic review. *J Hand Therapy.* 2021;34(1):3–17. https://doi.org/10.1016/j.jht.2020.05.003

9. Shepherd M, Louw A, Podolak J. The clinical application of pain neuroscience, graded motor imagery, and graded activity with complex regional pain syndrome-A case report. *Physiother Theory and Pract.* 2020;36(9):1043–1055. https://doi.org/10.1080/09593985.2018.1548047

10. Bailey KM, Carleton RN, Vlaeyen JW, Asmundson GJ. Treatments addressing pain-related fear and anxiety in patients with chronic musculoskeletal pain: A preliminary review. *Cogn Behav Ther.* 2010;39(1):46–63. https://doi.org/10.1080/16506070902980711

11. Chau B, Phelan I, Ta P, Chi B, Loyola K, Yeo E, et al. Immersive virtual reality for pain relief in upper limb complex regional pain syndrome: A pilot study. *Innov Clin Neurosci.* 2020;17(4–6):47–52.

12. Won AS, Barreau AC, Gaertner M, Stone T, Zhu J, Wang CY, et al. Assessing the feasibility of an open-source virtual reality mirror visual feedback module for complex regional pain syndrome: Pilot usability study. *J Med Internet Res.* 2021;23(5):e16536. https://doi.org/10.2196/16536

13. Moretti A, Palomba A, Paoletta M, Liguori S, Toro G, Iolascon G. Complex regional pain syndrome in athletes: Scoping review. *Medicina (Kaunas, Lithuania).* 2021;57(11):1262. https://doi.org/10.3390/medicina57111262

14. den Hollander M, Goossens M, de Jong J, Ruijgrok J, Oosterhof J, Onghena P, et al. Expose or protect? A randomized controlled trial of exposure in vivo vs pain-contingent treatment as usual in patients with complex regional pain syndrome type 1. *Pain.* 2016;157(10):2318–2329. https://doi.org/10.1097/j.pain.0000000000000651

15. Reeves L, Sako M, Malloy J, Goldstein A, Bennett K. Role of OT in comprehensive integrative pain management. AOTA. 2022. https://www.aota.org/practice/pract ice-essentials/quality/quality-resources/role-of-ot-pain-management

16. Oerlemans HM, Oostendorp RA, de Boo T, van der Laan L, Severens JL, Goris JA. Adjuvant physical therapy versus occupational therapy in patients with reflex sympathetic dystrophy/complex regional pain syndrome type I. *Arch Phys Med Rehabil*. 2000;81(1):49–56.

17. Waddell G, Newton M, Henderson I, Somerville D, Main CJ. A Fear-Avoidance Beliefs Questionnaire (FABQ) and the role of fear-avoidance beliefs in chronic low back pain and disability. *Pain*. 1993;52(2):157–168. https://doi.org/10.1016/0304-3959(93)90127-B

18. Boersma K, Linton SJ. Expectancy, fear and pain in the prediction of chronic pain and disability: A prospective analysis. *Eur J Pain (London)*. 2006;10(6):551–557. https://doi.org/10.1016/j.ejpain.2005.08.004

19. Harris S, Morley S, Barton SB. Role loss and emotional adjustment in chronic pain. *Pain*. 2003;105(1–2):363–370. https://doi.org/10.1016/s0304-3959(03)00251-3

20. Engel-Yeger B, Dunn W. Relationship between pain catastrophizing level and sensory processing patterns in typical adults. https://doi.org/10.5014/AJOT.2011.09004

21. Bar-Shalita T, Livshitz A, Levin-Meltz Y, Rand D, Deutsch L, Vatine JJ. Sensory modulation dysfunction is associated with complex regional pain syndrome. *PLOS ONE*. 2018;13(8):e0201354. https://doi.org/10.1371/journal.pone.0201354

22. Louw A, Zimney K, Puentedura EJ, Diener I. The efficacy of pain neuroscience education on musculoskeletal pain: A systematic review of the literature. *Physiother Theory Pract*. 2016;32(5):332–355. https://doi.org/10.1080/09593 985.2016.1194646

23. Antcliff D, Keenan AM, Keeley P, Woby S, McGowan L. Testing a newly developed activity pacing framework for chronic pain/fatigue: A feasibility study. *BMJ Open*. 2021;11(12):e045398. https://doi.org/10.1136/bmjopen-2020-045398

24. Moseley LG, Zalucki NM, Wiech K. Tactile discrimination, but not tactile stimulation alone, reduces chronic limb pain. *Pain*. 2008;137(3):600–608. https://doi.org/10.1016/j.pain.2007.10.021

25. Moseley LG, Wiech K. The effect of tactile discrimination training is enhanced when patients watch the reflected image of their unaffected limb during training. *Pain*. 2009;144(3):314–319. https://doi.org/10.1016/j.pain.2009.04.030

26. Horne CE, Engelke MK, Schreier A, Swanson M, Crane PB. Effects of tactile desensitization on postoperative pain after amputation surgery. *J Perianesthesia Nurs*. 2018;33(5):689–698. https://doi.org/10.1016/j.jopan.2017.02.005

27. Connelly JT. OTs role in cortical re-organization and resolving work-related CRPS type II. AOTA. 2020. https://www.aota.org/publications/sis-quarterly/work-indus try-sis/wisis-8-20

28. de Jong JR, Vlaeyen JWS, Onghena P, Cuypers C, den Hollander M, Ruijgrok J. Reduction of pain-related fear in complex regional pain syndrome type I: The application of graded exposure in vivo. *Pain*. 2005;116(3):264–275. https://doi.org/10.1016/j.pain.2005.04.019

29. van de Vusse AC, Stomp-van den Berg SG, Kessels AH, Weber WE. Randomised controlled trial of gabapentin in complex regional pain syndrome type 1 [ISRCTN84121379]. *BMC Neurol*. 2004;4:13. https://doi.org/10.1186/1471-2377-4-13

30. Javed S, Abdi S. Use of anticonvulsants and antidepressants for treatment of complex regional pain syndrome: A literature review. *Pain Manag*. 2021;11(2):189–199. https://doi.org/10.2217/pmt-2020-0060

31. Food and Drug Administration (FDA). FDA warns about serious breathing problems with seizure and nerve pain medicines gabapentin (Neurontin, Gralise, Horizant) and pregabalin (Lyrica, Lyrica CR). FDA. 2020. https://www.fda.gov/drugs/drug-safety-and-availability/fda-warns-about-serious-breathing-problems-seizure-and-nerve-pain-medicines-gabapentin-neurontin

32. Murnion BP. Neuropathic pain: Current definition and review of drug treatment. *Australian Prescriber*. 2018;41(3):60–63. https://doi.org/10.18773/austprescr.2018.022

33. Duong S, Bravo D, Todd KJ, Finlayson RJ, Tran Q. Treatment of complex regional pain syndrome: An updated systematic review and narrative synthesis. *Can J Anesth/Journal canadien danesthésie*. 2018;65(6):658–684. https://doi.org/10.1007/s12630-018-1091-5

34. Jamroz A, Berger M, Winston P. Prednisone for acute complex regional pain syndrome: A retrospective cohort study. *Pain Res Manag*. 2020:8182569. https://doi.org/10.1155/2020/8182569

35. Christensen K, Jensen EM, Noer I. The reflex dystrophy syndrome response to treatment with systemic corticosteroids. *Acta Chirurgica Scandi*. 1982;148(8):653–655.

36. Braus DF, Krauss JK, Strobel J. The shoulder–hand syndrome after stroke: A prospective clinical trial. *Ann Neurol*. 1994;36(5):728–733. https://doi.org/10.1002/ana.410360507

37. Kalita J, Vajpayee A, Misra UK. Comparison of prednisolone with piroxicam in complex regional pain syndrome following stroke: A randomized controlled trial. *QJM*. 2006;99(2):89–95. https://doi.org/10.1093/qjmed/hcl004

38. Breuer AJ, Mainka T, Hansel N, Maier C, Krumova EK. Short-term treatment with parecoxib for complex regional pain syndrome: A randomized, placebo-controlled double-blind trial. *Pain Physician*. 2014;17(2):127–137.

39. Harden RN, Oaklander AL, Burton AW, Perez RS, Richardson K, Swan M, et al. Complex regional pain syndrome: Practical diagnostic and treatment guidelines, 4th edition. *Pain Med(Malden, Mass.)*. 2013;14(2):180–229. https://doi.org/10.1111/pme.12033

40. Perez RS, Zollinger PE, Dijkstra PU, Thomassen-Hilgersom IL, Zuurmond WW, Rosenbrand KC, et al. Evidence based guidelines for complex regional pain syndrome type 1. *BMC Neurol*. 2010;10:20. https://doi.org/10.1186/1471-2377-10-20

41. Geertzen JH, de Bruijn H, de Bruijn-Kofman AT, Arendzen JH. Reflex sympathetic dystrophy: Early treatment and psychological aspects. *Arch Phys Med and Rehabil*. 1994;75(4):442–446. https://doi.org/10.1016/0003-9993(94)90169-4

42. Perez MRSG, Zuurmond AWW, Bezemer DP, Kuik JD, van Loenen CA, de Lange JJ, et al. The treatment of complex regional pain syndrome type I with free radical scavengers: A randomized controlled study. *Pain*. 2003;102(3):297–307. https://doi.org/10.1016/S0304-3959(02)00414-1

43. Yanow J, Pappagallo M, Pillai L. Complex regional pain syndrome (CRPS/RSD) and neuropathic pain: Role of intravenous bisphosphonates as analgesics. *Sci World J*. 2008;8:229–236. https://doi.org/10.1100/tsw.2008.33

44. Varenna M, Adami S, Sinigaglia L. Bisphosphonates in complex regional pain syndrome type I: How do they work?. *Clin Exp Rheumatol*. 2014;32(4):451–454.

45. Adami S, Fossaluzza V, Gatti D, Fracassi E, Braga V. Bisphosphonate therapy of reflex sympathetic dystrophy syndrome. *Ann Rheum Dis*. 1997;56(3):201–204. https://doi.org/10.1136/ard.56.3.201

46. Manicourt DH, Brasseur JP, Boutsen Y, Depreseux G, Devogelaer JP. Role of alendronate in therapy for posttraumatic complex regional pain syndrome type I of the lower extremity. *Arthritis Rheum*. 2004;50(11):3690–3697. https://doi.org/10.1002/art.20591

47. Varenna M, Zucchi F, Ghiringhelli D, Binelli L, Bevilacqua M, Bettica P, et al. Intravenous clodronate in the treatment of reflex sympathetic dystrophy syndrome. A randomized, double blind, placebo controlled study. *J Rheumatol*. 2000;27(6):1477–1483.

48. Varenna M, Adami S, Rossini M, Gatti D, Idolazzi L, Zucchi F, et al. Treatment of complex regional pain syndrome type I with neridronate: A randomized, double-blind, placebo-controlled study. *Rheumatology (Oxford, England)*. 2013;52(3):534–542. https://doi.org/10.1093/rheumatology/kes312

49. Robinson JN, Sandom J, Chapman PT. Efficacy of pamidronate in complex regional pain syndrome type I. *Pain Med (Malden, Mass.)*. 2004;5(3):276–280. https://doi.org/10.1111/j.1526-4637.2004.04038.x

50. Eun Young H, Hyeyun K, Sang Hee I. Pamidronate effect compared with a steroid on complex regional pain syndrome type I: Pilot randomised trial. *Netherlands J Med*. 2016;74(1):30–35.

51. Dunn KM, Saunders KW, Rutter CM, Banta-Green CJ, Merrill JO, Sullivan MD, et al. Opioid prescriptions for chronic pain and overdose: A cohort study. *Ann Intern Med*. 2010;152(2):85–92. https://doi.org/10.7326/0003-4819-152-2-201001190-00006

52. Chou R, Fanciullo GJ, Fine PG, Adler JA, Ballantyne JC, Davies P, et al. Clinical guidelines for the use of chronic opioid therapy in chronic noncancer pain. *J Pain*. 2009;10(2):113–130. https://doi.org/10.1016/j.jpain.2008.10.008

53. Descartes R. *De homine: Figuris et Latinitate donatus a Florentio Schuyl*. Apud Franciscum Moyardum & Petrum Leffen; 1662.

54. Flaten MA, al'Absi M. *Neuroscience of Pain, Stress, and Emotion: Psychological and Clinical Implications*. Academic Press; 2015.

55. Merskey H, Bogduk N. Part III: Pain terms, a current list with definitions and notes on usage. In *Classification of Chronic Pain, Second Edition, IASP Task Force on Taxonomy*. IASP Press; 2011:209–214.

56. Kosek E, Cohen M, Baron R, Gebhart GF, Mico JA, Rice ASC, et al. Do we need a third mechanistic descriptor for chronic pain states? *Pain*. 2016;157(7):1382–1386. https://doi.org/10.1097/j.pain.0000000000000507

57. Fitzcharles MA, Cohen SP, Clauw DJ, Littlejohn G, Usui C, Häuser W. Nociplastic pain: Towards an understanding of prevalent pain conditions. *Lancet (London)*. 2021;397(10289):2098–2110. https://doi.org/10.1016/S0140-6736(21)00392-5

58. Siddall PJ. Neuroplasticity and pain: What does it all mean? *Med J Australia*. 2013;198(4):177–178. https://doi.org/10.5694/mja13.10100

59. Kuner R, Flor H. Structural plasticity and reorganisation in chronic pain. *Nat Rev Neurosci*. 2016;18(1):20–30. https://doi.org/10.1038/nrn.2016.162

60. Melzack R, Wall PD. Pain mechanisms: A new theory. *Science*. 1965;150(3699):971–979. https://doi.org/10.1126/science.150.3699.971

61. Zhang L, Lu X, Bi Y, Hu L. Pavlov's pain: The effect of classical conditioning on pain perception and its clinical implications. *Curr Pain Headache Rep*. 2019;23(3):19. https://doi.org/10.1007/s11916-019-0766-0

62. Sullivan MJ, Thorn B, Haythornthwaite JA, Keefe F, Martin M, Bradley LA, et al. Theoretical perspectives on the relation between catastrophizing and pain. *Clin J Pain*. 2001;17(1):52–64. https://doi.org/10.1097/00002508-200103000-00008

63. Im JJ, Kim J, Jeong H, Oh JK, Lee S, Lyoo IK, et al. Prefrontal white matter abnormalities associated with pain catastrophizing in patients with complex regional pain syndrome. *Arch Phys Med Rehabil*. 2021;102(2):216–224. https://doi.org/10.1016/j.apmr.2020.07.006

64. Moseley GL, Vlaeyen JWS. Beyond nociception: The imprecision hypothesis of chronic pain. *Pain*. 2015;156(1):35–38. https://doi.org/10.1016/j.pain.0000000000000014

65. Holmes A, Christelis N, Arnold C. Depression and chronic pain. *Med J Australia*. 2013;199(S6):S17–20. https://doi.org/10.5694/mja12.10589

66. Bass C, Yates G. Complex regional pain syndrome type 1 in the medico-legal setting: High rates of somatoform disorders, opiate use and diagnostic uncertainty. *Med Sci Law*. 2018;58(3):147–155. https://doi.org/10.1177/0025802418779934

67. Feldman SI, Downey G, Schaffer-Neitz R. Pain, negative mood, and perceived support in chronic pain patients: A daily diary study of people with reflex sympathetic dystrophy syndrome. *J Consult Clin Psychol.* 1999;67(5):776–785. https://doi.org/10.1037//0022-006x.67.5.776

68. Turk DC, Okifuji A. Psychological factors in chronic pain: Evolution and revolution. *J Consult Clin Psychol.* 2002;70(3):678–690. https://doi.org/10.1037//0022-006x.70.3.678

69. Speck V, Schlereth T, Birklein F, Maihöfner C. Increased prevalence of posttraumatic stress disorder in CRPS. *Eur J Pain (London).* 2017;21(3):466–473. https://doi.org/10.1002/ejp.940

70. Morley S, Eccleston C, Williams A. Systematic review and meta-analysis of randomized controlled trials of cognitive behaviour therapy and behaviour therapy for chronic pain in adults, excluding headache. *Pain.* 1999;80(1–2):1–13. https://doi.org/10.1016/s0304-3959(98)00255-3

71. Hughes LS, Clark J, Colclough JA, Dale E, McMillan D. Acceptance and Commitment Therapy (ACT) for chronic pain: A systematic review and meta-analyses. *Clin J Pain.* 2017;33(6):552–568. https://doi.org/10.1097/AJP.0000000000000425

72. Cho S, McCracken LM, Heiby EM, Moon DE, Lee JH. Pain acceptance-based coping in complex regional pain syndrome Type I: Daily relations with pain intensity, activity, and mood. *J Behav Med.* 2013;36(5):531–538. https://doi.org/10.1007/s10865-012-9448-7

73. Hudson J, Lake E, Spruit E, Terrell M, Cooper K, McFawn C. Comprehensive rehabilitation of patients with complex regional pain syndrome. Complex Regional Pain Syndrome. 2021. https://doi.org/10.1007/978-3-030-75373-3_7

5   Modulate, Reset, Intervene

Yan Yin and Jianguo Cheng

Case

A 23-year-old female athlete was diagnosed with
complex regional pain syndrome (CRPS) type I in her
left leg after twisting her left ankle 6 months ago. The
pain, together with swelling, redness, and extreme
sensitivity to touch, remains unbearable despite
physical therapy and multiple oral analgesics for
the past several months. She is interested in some
advanced techniques that may help relieve her pain
but is not ready yet for any implants in her body.

What Do I Do Now?

INTERVENTIONAL TREATMENTS AS PART
OF MULTIMODAL THERAPY

The optimal approach to complex regional pain syndrome (CRPS) treatment is multimodal and comprehensive. Previous chapters have discussed pharmacotherapy and physical therapy. Interventional therapies, such as sympathetic or peripheral nerve blocks, also have long held a role in pain relief depending on whether the pain is sympathetically mediated pain (SMP) or sympathetically independent pain (SIP). These techniques facilitate physical therapy and may reduce the pain to a level that cannot be achieved with oral analgesics. In addition, intravenous infusion of different classes of medications, including but not limited to ketamine, sympatholytic agents, anti-inflammatory medications, and other N-methyl-D-aspartate (NMDA) receptor antagonists, has been investigated as a treatment for CRPS.[1] The rationale of using these agents is that enhanced sympathetic tone, NMDA signaling activation, and undue inflammatory reaction in the nervous system may play a critical role in the pathogenesis of CRPS. We recently provided more comprehensive reviews of interventional management[2] and infusion therapies for CRPS.[1]

SYMPATHETIC BLOCKS

One of the most commonly described procedures in the management of CRPS is a sympathetic block utilized for diagnostic and therapeutic purposes. Perturbations in the sympathetic nervous system have been implicated as an important mechanism in CRPS. In the afferent pathways, such blocks aim to disrupt nociceptive as well as visceral and somatic afferent fibers. In addition, blockade of sudomotor, visceromotor, and vasomotor efferent fibers may be therapeutic for symptoms of CRPS. Most algorithms advocate sympathetic blocks to distinguish between SMP and SIP, which may have treatment implications.[3] A systematic review evaluating sympathetic blocks for CRPS found scant evidence for meaningful therapeutic benefit based on predominantly low-quality studies.[4] However, in a more recent study, we demonstrated substantial evidence for clinically meaningful pain reduction in the majority of a large cohort of patients with CRPS.[5] This finding is further supported by a recently published randomized controlled trial demonstrating that lumbar sympathetic block with botulinum toxin A reduced pain and increased limb temperature for 3 months.[6]

The sympathetic blocks used for CRPS are stellate ganglion block (SGB), upper thoracic sympathetic block, and lumbar sympathetic block (LSB). Blocking the stellate ganglion, which is located anterior to the C6–7 transverse processes, is used for CRPS in the upper extremity. The block can be performed by landmark-based technique, under fluoroscopy, CT, or ultrasound guidance. Fluoroscopy and ultrasound guidance are the most commonly used approaches. Under fluoroscopy guidance in oblique view, a needle is inserted at the junction of the transverse process and corresponding C6 or C7 vertebral body. Contact is made with bone and an anteroposterior view is obtained by fluoroscopy to assess needle position. Once needle position is adequate, 0.5–1 mL of contrast dye is injected to confirm correct needle tip position and to prevent intravascular or another off-target injection. The contrast dye should spread over the prevertebral sympathetic chain at C6–T1. Thereafter, SGB is performed with injection of local anesthetic (often 1% lidocaine or 0.25% bupivacaine) or a combination of local anesthetic and steroid (dexamethasone 10 mg, for instance) to prolong the blockade. Botulinum toxin A has also been used. When clinically indicated, neurolysis of the stellate ganglion can be performed using radiofrequency ablation. The specific radiofrequency protocol may differ among institutions. In contrast to fluoroscopy, ultrasound imaging aims to identify the prevertebral fascia and allow for the precise deposition of the injectate between the longus colli muscle and longus capitis muscle. Proponents of this approach argue that ultrasound guidance reduces x-ray exposure and increases the specificity of the procedure in blocking the sympathetic chain alone. Bilateral SGB performed on the same day should be avoided to prevent bilateral recurrent laryngeal nerve block and the consequent vocal cord paralysis and respiratory compromise.

In some patients, SGB alone may not achieve sufficient sympatholysis in the upper extremity. This might be due to the direct projection of thoracic sympathetic ganglia to the brachial plexus, bypassing the cervical or stellate ganglia. In this case, a thoracic sympathetic block at T2 level can be performed. This procedure is technically challenging due to risks of pneumothorax and should be performed under fluoroscopy or CT guidance by experienced clinicians.

The LSB has been widely used to manage CRPS pain in the lower extremity. It is performed under fluoroscopy, CT, or ultrasound image guidance. The lumbar sympathetic ganglia, the convergence of pre- and post-ganglionic fibers, are located at the anterolateral side of the L2–4 lumbar vertebrae. Under fluoroscopic anteroposterior view, the L3 level is identified with the patient in the prone position. At oblique view and using sterile technique, the skin is infiltrated with local anesthetic and then a needle is advanced toward the anterolateral edge of the target T2 or T3 lumbar vertebra. The lateral view is then obtained to confirm needle tip in the anterolateral edge of the target lumbar vertebra, with final position confirmed with contrast dye injection. The contrast dye should outline over the prevertebral sympathetic chain at L2–4. Finally, local anesthetic is injected. A local anesthetic blockade may be followed-up, if clinically indicated, with a more definitive block using radiofrequency ablation. The use of botulinum toxin has also been reported to prolong the blockade and therapeutic effects.[6,7]

Sympathetic blocks are performed with injection of local anesthetic (often 1% lidocaine or 0.25% bupivacaine). The blocks are usually effective in reducing CRPS pain, but the efficacy is often short-lived, a matter of hours. A combination of local anesthetic and steroid (dexamethasone 10 mg, for instance) is commonly used to prolong the blockade to a few days or a few weeks. The use of botulinum toxin for LSB may prolong the analgesic effect to 3 months.[6,7] Chemical or thermal neurolysis of lumbar sympathetic ganglion has largely fallen out of favor due to untoward complications.

Change in limb temperature after sympathetic block has been used to confirm a technically successful blockade. In a large retrospective cohort study, we found that sympathetic blocks may be therapeutic in patients with CRPS regardless of pre- and post-procedure limb temperatures.[5] We also found that the effects of sympathetic blocks do not predict the success of spinal cord stimulation. Interestingly, in a multicenter study, we found that the response to sympathetic blocks may predict response to ketamine infusion in CRPS patients, with alleviation of the affective component of pain.[8]

PERIPHERAL NERVE BLOCKS

CRPS patients with SIP who do not respond to sympathetic blocks may respond to a combined somatic/sympathetic block.[9] Like sympathetic blocks, these blocks can be performed as a series of blocks or make use of an indwelling catheter as a continuous block. Continuous peripheral nerve blocks through a catheter (0.1 mL/kg/h ropivacaine, 0.2%, for 96 hours) using an elastomeric pump after a 20-minute Bier block (0.2 mL/kg lido-caine, 1%; 3 mL/kg hydroxyethyl starch 130/06; and 5 mg/kg buflomedil) were performed in 13 pediatric patients.[10] All patients were followed-up after 2 months. Ambulatory continuous peripheral nerve block provided significant pain relief, early mobilization, and rapid return home. Epidural block through a dwelling tunneled catheter can be effective for CRPS, but infections, particularly epidural space infections, have been a concern.[11]

INTRAVENOUS THERAPIES

Our systematic review concluded that there is some evidence to support the use of intravenous bisphosphonates, immunoglobulin, ketamine, or lido-caine as valuable interventions in selected patients with CRPS.[1] However, high-quality studies are required to further evaluate the safety, efficacy, and cost-effectiveness of intravenous therapies for CRPS.

INTRAVENOUS KETAMINE INFUSION

Ketamine intravenous infusion to block NMDA signaling and central sen-sitization has been used to manage intractable CRPS pain, particularly in patients who have failed to respond to other therapies such as nerve blocks and spinal cord stimulation. There is weak evidence, based on low-quality studies, for benefit lasting more than 4 weeks. Our recent multicenter study demonstrated that ketamine infusion achieved a 61% success rate in reducing CRPS-related pain by greater than 30% for more than 4 weeks in patients with SMP, while the success rate was reduced to 27% in patients with SIP.[8] One of the challenges with ketamine infusion is the wide variation in treatment protocols in terms of dosage, infusion duration, infusion frequency, patient selection, and outcomes measurement. A consensus protocol of ketamine infusion for CRPS has been suggested by a panel of experts but has yet to be validated.[12]

Bier Block

The intravenous regional anesthesia, or Bier block, injects local anesthetic into a peripheral vein of an upper or lower extremity that has been exsanguinated by compression or gravity and that has been isolated by means of a tourniquet from the central circulation. It is often uncomfortable for patients with CRPS. Its use is, therefore, limited to certain patients who can tolerate the pneumonic tourniquet. Case reports showed that Bier block could be an option in refractory CRPS. A patient with CRPS in the upper extremity had only 1 week of relief after SGB or pulsed radiofrequency ablation of the stellate ganglion and failed brachial plexus block. A Bier block (20 mL lidocaine 0.5% and 8 mg dexamethasone) provided the patient remarkable pain relief for 6 months.[13] Another patient with CRPS in the leg did not respond to a standard Bier block with bretylium and lidocaine but responded for 7 years to multiple Bier blocks with labetalol and lidocaine.[14] However, a randomized, double-blinded, placebo-controlled trial found that Bier block with methylprednisolone and lidocaine did not provide long-term benefit in CRPS, and its short-term benefit was not superior to placebo.[15] The most worrisome complication of Bier block is local anesthetic systemic toxicity. Careful calculation of the maximum dose and correct use of the tourniquet are key measures to minimize the incidence of this complication.

For the patient described in our case study, we would first recommend LSB for her CRPS pain in the lower extremity. If pain relief is insufficient from LSB, we would recommend neuromodulation with dorsal root ganglion stimulation or spinal cord stimulation. If the patient is not interested in neuromodulation or fails to respond to neuromodulation, we would recommend intravenous ketamine infusion or Bier block.

- Sympathetic blocks, such as stellate ganglion block (SGB), upper thoracic sympathetic block, and lumbar sympathetic block (LSB), could be effective for sympathetically mediated pain in complex regional pain syndrome (CRPS).
- For sympathetically independent pain in CRPS, peripheral nerve blocks with or without an indwelling catheter can be considered.
- Intravenous ketamine infusion or Bier block can be considered for CRPS pain relief if the patient has failed other therapies or is not interested in neuromodulation.

Suggested Reading

Carroll I, Clark JD, Mackey S. Sympathetic block with botulinum toxin to treat complex regional pain syndrome. *Ann Neurol.* 2009;65:348–351.

Cheng J, Salmasi V, You J, Grille M, Yang D, Mascha EJ, et al. Outcomes of sympathetic blocks in the management of complex regional pain syndrome: A retrospective cohort study. *Anesthesiology.* 2019;131:883–893.

Cohen SP, Khunsriraksakul C, Yoo Y, Parker E, Samen-Akinsiku CDK, Patel N, et al. Sympathetic blocks as a predictor for response to ketamine infusion in patients with complex regional pain syndrome: A multicenter study. *Pain Med.* 2022.

References

1. Xu J, Yang J, Lin P, Rosenquist E, Cheng J. Intravenous therapies for complex regional pain syndrome: A systematic review. *Anesth Analg.* 2016;122:843–856.
2. Shin, C, Cheng J. Interventional treatments for CRPS. In Lawson E, Castellanos J, eds. *Complex Regional Pain Syndrome.* Springer Nature; 2021.
3. Harden RN, Oaklander AL, Burton AW, Perez RS, Richardson K, Swan M, et al. Complex regional pain syndrome: Practical diagnostic and treatment guidelines, 4th edition. *Pain Med.* 2013;14:180–229.
4. O'Connell NE, Wand BM, Gibson W, Carr DB, Birklein F, Stanton TR. Local anaesthetic sympathetic blockade for complex regional pain syndrome. *Cochrane Database Syst Rev.* 2016;7:Cd004598.
5. Cheng J, Salmasi V, You J, Grille M, Yang D, Mascha EJ, et al. Outcomes of sympathetic blocks in the management of complex regional pain syndrome: A retrospective cohort study. *Anesthesiology.* 2019;131:883–893.
6. Yoo Y, Lee CS, Kim J, Jo D, Moon JY. Botulinum toxin type A for lumbar sympathetic ganglion block in complex regional pain syndrome: A randomized trial. *Anesthesiology.* 2022;136:314–325.

7. Carroll I, Clark JD, Mackey S. Sympathetic block with botulinum toxin to treat complex regional pain syndrome. *Ann Neurol.* 2009;65:348–351.
8. Cohen SP, Khunsriraksakul C, Yoo Y, Parker E, Samen-Akinsiku CDK, Patel N, et al. Sympathetic blocks as a predictor for response to ketamine infusion in patients with complex regional pain syndrome: A multicenter study. *Pain Med.* 2022.
9. Rho RH, Brewer RP, Lamer TJ, Wilson PR. Complex regional pain syndrome. *Mayo Clin Proc.* 2002;77:174–180.
10. Dadure C, Motais F, Ricard C, Raux O, Troncin R, Capdevila X. Continuous peripheral nerve blocks at home for treatment of recurrent complex regional pain syndrome I in children. *Anesthesiology.* 2005;102:387–391.
11. Hayek SM, Paige B, Girgis G, Kapural L, Fattouh M, Xu M, et al. Tunneled epidural catheter infections in noncancer pain: Increased risk in patients with neuropathic pain/complex regional pain syndrome. *Clin J Pain.* 2006;22:82–89.
12. Xu J, Herndon C, Anderson S, Getson P, Foorsov V, Harbut RE, et al. Intravenous ketamine infusion for complex regional pain syndrome: Survey, consensus, and a reference protocol. *Pain Med,* 2019;20:323–334.
13. Emami SA, Majedi H, Espahbodi E, Sanatkar M. Bier block as a successful management of a patient with intractable complex regional pain syndrome (CRPS) type 1: A case report. *Clin Case Rep.* 2021;9:e04554.
14. Hord ED, Stojanovic MP, Vallejo R, Barna SA, Santiago-Palma J, Mao J. Multiple Bier blocks with labetalol for complex regional pain syndrome refractory to other treatments. *J Pain Symptom Manag.* 2003;25:299–302.
15. Taskaynatan MA, Ozgul A, Tan AK, Dincer K, Kalyon TA. Bier block with methylprednisolone and lidocaine in CRPS type I: A randomized, double-blinded, placebo-controlled study. *Reg Anesth Pain Med.* 2004;29:408–412.

Breaking Up the Signal

Justin C. Grubbs, Jonathan W. Kim, and
Lawrence R. Poree

Case

A 42-year-old woman presents to the clinic with a
right-sided foot injury from a mechanical fall 1 year
ago. The wound was sutured in the emergency room,
and she was followed by podiatry for ongoing foot
pain. Since the injury, she endorses worsening whole
foot pain with redness, swelling, and increased
temperature. An MRI of the foot shows no neuroma
or severe pathology to explain her widespread
symptoms. Physical therapy, gabapentin, and topical
ointments have not been helpful. She has seen a pain
physician who performed three lumbar sympathetic
blocks resulting in only temporary and minor relief.
On physical exam, her right foot is edematous,
erythematous, and sensitive to light touch. She has
decreased range of motion in her right ankle and has
difficulty bearing weight on this side.

What Do I Do Now?

WHEN CONSERVATIVE TREATMENT FAILS

Complex regional pain syndrome (CRPS) is often unresponsive and has the potential to become resistant to conservative treatment modalities, especially when it is chronic in nature.[1] Therefore, it has become common international practice to use spinal cord stimulation (SCS) to treat CRPS when other modalities fail to provide pain relief, quality of life, or improvement in function.[2]

PROCEDURE

SCS is a form of spinal neuromodulation analgesia and involves application of electrical stimulation to the nervous system.[3] It is used for chronic pain from nervous system injury that has failed conservative management. It is both minimally invasive and reversible, and it involves percutaneously or surgically implanting electrodes into the epidural space to generate an electrical field over the spinal dorsal column. A temporary screening trial is conducted with an external pulse generator connected to the electrodes to assess efficacy and adverse effects. On average, the screening trial lasts 4–10 days. The trial is generally considered successful if greater than 50% pain reduction occurs with improved functionality. If the trial is successful, implantation is then recommended.[4]

The SCS system generates a weak electrical field to stimulate the spinal cord's dorsal column. This may evoke peripheral paresthesias in the corresponding dermatomes. Implantation may be performed under local anesthesia in order to utilize patient feedback regarding the coverage of these paresthesias. If the provider can achieve complete or near-complete overlap between the source of the patient's pain and the location of the evoked paresthesias, optimal electrode placement is ensured, with resultant pain relief once the device is active. After implantation, the provider can program the device to no longer elicit paresthesias.[1]

Initially, the hypothesis of analgesia from SCS was thought to be consistent with the gate control theory in the dorsal horn of the spinal cord. However, newer theories demonstrate that SCS may also treat neuropathic pain in part by wide dynamic range neuron suppression in the dorsal horn or inhibition of glial cells. Pain relief from SCS may take days to weeks to achieve effect, which points to a central mechanism of analgesia.[4]

SCS may play a role in modulating the inflammatory aspect of CRPS, which contributes to pain, swelling, and warmth. Kriek et al. showed that, after SCS implantation, the expression of both pro- and anti-inflammatory cytokines decreased over time in both the affected and unaffected extremities.[5] SCS was found to attenuate T-cell activation, improve peripheral tissue oxygenation, and decrease anti-angiogenetic activity. This then leads to diminished endothelial dysfunction and improved blood flow.

Common indications for SCS include thoracic and lumbar post-laminectomy syndrome ("failed back surgery syndrome"), refractory radiculitis of the upper or lower extremity, CRPS, HIV polyneuropathy, diabetic neuropathy, pain from epidural fibrosis, and pain from arachnoiditis. In Europe, SCS is more commonly used for intractable angina and peripheral vascular disease.[4]

OUTCOMES

SCS has demonstrated efficacy in treating CRPS type I. Eriksen et al. conducted a retrospective cohort study to assess the long-term effect of SCS on multiple outcomes in a cohort of CRPS patients.[1] Their study of 51 patients demonstrated a significant effect on pain relief with a mean reduction in the numeric rating scale (NRS) score of 2.4 (95% confidence interval [CI]: 1.7–3.0, $p < 0.0001$). Of note, the mean NRS score remained significantly reduced through 8 years of follow-up. When assessing the Patients' Global Impression of Change, 68.8% of participants reported to be "much improved" or "very much improved." Of the participants, 87.5% reported they would choose to have the SCS implanted again for the same outcome. Improved symptoms of depression, decreased pain catastrophizing, improved quality of life, and decreased consumption of other analgesics (tricyclic antidepressants, antiepileptic drugs, and opioids) were other measured outcomes that revealed significant benefit with the use of SCS.

However, other research suggests diminishing pain-alleviating effects of SCS with time.[6,7] A prospective, randomized trial of 54 patients with CRPS type I conducted by Kemler et al. randomized patients to SCS with physical therapy or physical therapy alone, with two-thirds in the SCS arm going on to implantation.[8] At 6 months, pain was reduced in the SCS arm by 2.4 cm on a 10-cm visual analogue scale of pain intensity compared to a 0.2 cm increase in the control group. Also, 39% of patients in the SCS group rated their pain as "much improved" compared to 6% in the control group. Both cervical and lumbar devices were found to be effective. At 2 years post-implantation, CRPS patients continued to report efficacy from SCS. However, a 5-year follow-up study revealed diminishing effectiveness of SCS over time, after about 3 years of therapy.[7] This phenomenon of loss of efficacy despite initial success, known as *habituation*, is not completely understood and is one of the most common causes of hardware removal.[9,10] Despite the diminishing effect, patient satisfaction from those with SCS remained high, and more than 95% of patients with an implant reported they would repeat the treatment for the same results.[7]

Overall, research regarding SCS in the treatment of CRPS has provided high-level evidence (1B+) to support its role in improving CRPS patients' pain and quality of life.[2] Additionally, an independent systematic review concluded that there was evidence that SCS used to treat CRPS type I demonstrated efficacy relative to conventional medical management.[11] However, the European Federation of Neurological Societies gave a weak recommendation for the use of SCS for CRPS type I given the moderate amount of quality evidence.[12] Furthermore, to date, there is a lack of evidence to support SCS efficacy for patients with CRPS type II.[10] Overall, more research needs to be done to further elucidate the possible role of SCS in resolving CRPS signs and improving functional status, sleep, psychological impacts, and measures of analgesic-sparing effects.

COMPLICATIONS

While SCS offers numerous therapeutic benefits, it is not without its risks. Potential complications arising from SCS implantation include:

- *Lead migration* (13.2%): This can result in inadequate paresthesia coverage, leading to diminished pain relief. Reprogramming may address the issue in most cases. However, surgical correction becomes necessary in 16–23% of such situations to ensure optimal paresthesia coverage.[13]

- *Lead fracture* (9.1%), *loose connection* (0.4%), *hardware malfunction* (2.9%): These equipment-related complications typically necessitate surgical revision.[13]
- *Infection* (3.4%): Superficial infections can be treated with antibiotics, but if the infection is deeper, explantation becomes necessary.[14] Early recognition and treatment are crucial because untreated infections can become life-threatening. One case report cited a patient developing paralysis due to an infection at the lead tip.[13] Therefore, screening for infection risk factors, such as diabetes mellitus, preexisting infections, poor hygiene, malnutrition, and corticosteroid use, is essential and should be managed prior to implantation.[14]
- *Dural puncture* (0.3%): Accidental dural punctures can result in postdural puncture headaches from cerebral spinal fluid leakage. While small dural punctures typically heal spontaneously, persistent headaches can be addressed with an epidural blood patch.[13]
- *Epidural hematoma* (0.3%): This is generally deemed an emergency warranting immediate medical intervention.[4]
- *Paralysis* (0.03%): Though exceedingly rare, paralysis can result from SCS complications, as described earlier.[13]

Additionally, as mentioned previously, habituation is a known treatment-limiting complication of SCS resulting in reduced efficacy over time and has been observed in 41% of all explants.[9,10]

Most complications are not life-threatening and are reversible. However, their potential implications underscore the importance of thorough patient evaluation, meticulous surgical technique, and attentive postoperative care.

SUMMARY

SCS should be reserved for CRPS patients who do not respond to conservative treatments or who are candidates for sympathetic nerve blocks. Many studies show significant benefit in the first 2–3 years that tends to wane due to habituation. Despite this effect, patient satisfaction remains high, and SCS should be considered if patients are afflicted with refractory CRPS.

- Spinal cord stimulation (SCS) can be beneficial in the treatment of complex regional pain syndrome (CRPS) type I.
- SCS works by treating neuropathic pain and may modulate the inflammatory response in CRPS.
- SCS should be considered for patients with CRPS and refractory to conservative treatments.
- Numerous studies demonstrate waning efficacy over time for some patients, a process known as *habituation.*
- Despite habituation from SCS, long-term studies demonstrate high patient satisfaction.
- Careful selection of the appropriate patient for SCS therapy is critical given the associated risks.

Suggested Reading

Eriksen LE, Terkelsen AJ, Blichfeldt-Eckhardt MR, Sørensen JCH, Meier K. Spinal cord stimulation in severe cases of complex regional pain syndrome: A retrospective cohort study with long-term follow-up. *Eur J Pain (London).* 2021;25(10):2212–2225. https://doi.org/10.1002/ejp.1834

Stanton-Hicks M. 2006. Complex regional pain syndrome: Manifestations and the role of neurostimulation in its management. *J Pain Sympt Manag.* 2006;31(4 Suppl):S20–S24. https://doi.org/10.1016/j.jpainsymman.2005.12.011

Visnjevac O, Costandi S, Patel BA, Azer G, Agarwal P, Bolash R, Mekhail NA. 2017. A comprehensive outcome-specific review of the use of spinal cord stimulation for complex regional pain syndrome. *Pain Pract.* 2017;17(4):533–545. https://doi.org/10.1111/papr.12513

References

1. Eriksen LE, Terkelsen AJ, Blichfeldt-Eckhardt MR, Sørensen JCH, Meier K. Spinal cord stimulation in severe cases of complex regional pain syndrome: A retrospective cohort study with long-term follow-up. *Eur J Pain (London).* 2021;25 (10):2212–2225. https://doi.org/10.1002/ejp.1834

2. Visnjevac O, Costandi S, Patel BA, Azer G, Agarwal P, Bolash R, Mekhail NA. A comprehensive outcome-specific review of the use of spinal cord stimulation for complex regional pain syndrome. *Pain Pract.* 2017;17(4):533–545. https://doi.org/10.1111/papr.12513

3. Stanton-Hicks M. Complex regional pain syndrome: Manifestations and the role of neurostimulation in its management. *J Pain Sympt Manag*. 2006;31(4 Suppl):S20–S24. https://doi.org/10.1016/j.jpainsymman.2005.12.011

4. Sabia M, Mathur R. *Interventional Pain Procedures: Handbook and Video Guide* (1st ed.). Demos Medical; 2018.

5. Kriek N, Schreurs MWJ, Groeneweg JG, Dik WA, Tjiang GCH, Gültuna I, et al. Spinal cord stimulation in patients with complex regional pain syndrome: A possible target for immunomodulation? *Neuromodulation*. 2018;21(1):77–86. https://doi.org/10.1111/ner.12704

6. Geurts JW, Smits H, Kemler MA, Brunner F, Kessels AGH, van Kleef M. Spinal cord stimulation for complex regional pain syndrome type I: A prospective cohort study with long-term follow-up. *Neuromodulation*. 2013;16 (6):523–529; discussion 529. https://doi.org/10.1111/ner.12024

7. Kemler MA, De Vet HCW Barendse GAM, Van Den Wildenberg FAJM, Van Kleef M. Effect of spinal cord stimulation for chronic complex regional pain syndrome type I: Five-year final follow-up of patients in a randomized controlled trial. *J Neurosurg*. 2008;108(2):292–298. https://doi.org/10.3171/JNS/2008/108/2/0292

8. Kemler MA, De Vet HCW Barendse GAM, Van Den Wildenberg FAJM, Van Kleef M. The effect of spinal cord stimulation in patients with chronic reflex sympathetic dystrophy: Two years' follow-up of the randomized controlled trial. *Ann Neurol*. 2004;55(1):13–18. https://doi.org/10.1002/ana.10996

9. Hayek SM, Veizi E, Hanes M. Treatment-limiting complications of percutaneous spinal cord stimulator implants: A review of eight years of experience from an academic center database. *Neuromodulation*. 2015;18(7):603–608; discussion 608–609. https://doi.org/10.1111/ner.12312

10. Dworkin RH, O'Connor AB, Kent J, Mackey SC, Raja SN, Stacey BR, Levy RM, et al. Interventional management of neuropathic pain: NeuPSIG recommendations. *Pain*. 2013;154(11):2249–2261. https://doi.org/10.1016/j.pain.2013.06.004

11. Simpson EL, Duenas A, Holmes MW, Papaioannou D, Chilcott J. Spinal cord stimulation for chronic pain of neuropathic or ischaemic origin: Systematic review and economic evaluation. *Health Technol Assess (Winchester, England)*. 2009;13(17):iii, ix–x, 1–154. https://doi.org/10.3310/hta13170

12. Cruccu G, Aziz TZ, Garcia-Larrea L, Hansson P, Jensen TS, Lefaucheur J-P, Simpson BA, Taylor RS. EFNS guidelines on neurostimulation therapy for neuropathic pain. *Eur J Neurol*. 2007;14(9):952–970. https://doi.org/10.1111/j.1468-1331.2007.01916.x

13. Cameron T. Safety and efficacy of spinal cord stimulation for the treatment of chronic pain: A 20-year literature review. *J Neurosurg*. 2004;100(3 Suppl Spine):254–267. https://doi.org/10.3171/spi.2004.100.3.0254

14. Follett KA, Boortz-Marx RL, Drake JM, DuPen S, Schneider SJ, Turner MS, Coffey RJ. Prevention and management of intrathecal drug delivery and spinal cord stimulation system infections. *Anesthesiology*. 2004;100(6):1582–1594. https://doi.org/10.1097/00000542-200406000-00034

A New Target

Shrif Costandi, Kerolous Eldeeb, Youstina Bolok, and Samuel Samuel

Case

A 30-year-old man presents with chronic pain in the left ankle following a machine injury. The patient had undergone five corrective surgeries over 12 months. On exam, the patient exhibited allodynia and decreased range of motion of the ankle along with left foot nail trophic changes. Purple discoloration and swelling of the left foot were seen on the exam. The right foot was normal. The patient was diagnosed with complex regional pain syndrome (CRPS) type I and was started on opioids and oral steroids without any alleviation of pain or other symptoms. Pregabalin was added to his regimen without any benefit. Moreover, the patient suffered from drowsiness from his oral analgesics. The patient failed to respond to multiple sessions of physical therapy and wanted to discuss a novel nerve root stimulation therapy.

What Do I Do Now?

NEUROMODULATION FOR REFRACTORY COMPLEX REGIONAL PAIN SYNDROME

Complex regional pain syndrome (CRPS) is a condition affecting an extremity, usually following an injury. Patients usually complain of prolonged pain or inflammation without resolution of symptoms despite multiple therapies. CRPS management includes topical and oral medications, sympathetic block and neurolysis, and spinal cord stimulation (SCS) (please refer to previous chapters).

SCS and dorsal root ganglion (DRG) stimulation[1] are two neuromodulation techniques used to manage complex regional pain syndrome (CRPS). While both methods have shown efficacy in treating CRPS, they have differences in their mechanisms of action and clinical applications. A comparison of spinal cord stimulation (SCS) and DRG stimulation for CRPS includes:

- *Targeted area*: SCS involves the placement of electrodes in the epidural space over the dorsal columns of the spinal cord. It primarily targets the spinal cord to modulate pain signals. DRG stimulation targets specific dorsal root ganglia (DRG), which are located near the spinal cord and are responsible for transmitting sensory signals from peripheral nerves to the spinal cord. DRG stimulation directly influences these sensory pathways.
- *Mechanism of action*: SCS works by electrically stimulating the spinal cord to interfere with the transmission of pain signals to the brain. It generates paresthesia (tingling sensation) in the painful area, which can mask the perception of pain. DRG stimulation selectively stimulates the DRG associated with the affected limb or body region. It modulates pain signals at their source, affecting sensory neurons before they reach the spinal cord.
- *Paresthesia*: Typically, SCS induces paresthesia, which some patients may find uncomfortable or unpleasant. Paresthesia coverage needs to be precisely adjusted to target the painful area effectively. DRG stimulation can be programmed to provide paresthesia-free stimulation. This makes it a suitable option for patients who are sensitive to paresthesia or have discomfort with traditional SCS.

- *Pain relief:* SCS has been used successfully for CRPS pain management, offering relief to many patients (see Chapter 6). However, the degree of pain relief can vary among individuals. DRG stimulation has shown promise as a targeted therapy for CRPS, and some studies suggest that it may provide more precise and effective pain relief, especially for distal extremity CRPS.
- *Implantation site:* In SCS, electrodes are placed in the epidural space, and the generator is usually implanted in the upper buttock or abdominal region. In DRG stimulation, electrodes are placed directly at the DRG site near the spinal cord. The generator is typically implanted near the targeted DRG.
- *Patient selection:* SCS is often considered for CRPS patients with pain affecting broader areas, such as the trunk or multiple extremities. DRG stimulation may be particularly beneficial for patients with focal or distal extremity CRPS.

In summary, both SCS and DRG stimulation have shown effectiveness in managing CRPS, but they differ in their mechanisms of action and suitability for specific patient profiles. The choice between the two should be made based on individual patient characteristics, pain distribution, and response to paresthesia-based or paresthesia-free stimulation. Consulting with a pain management specialist is essential to determine the most appropriate treatment approach for each CRPS patient.

EFFICACY OF DORSAL ROOT GANGLION STIMULATION FOR CRPS

The ACCURATE study, a controlled, randomized, multicenter study evaluated the safety and efficacy of DRG stimulation compared to traditional SCS for CRPS in the lower extremity.[2] The percentage of patients reporting greater than 50% pain relief was greater in the DRG group (81.2%, $n = 61$) compared to the SCS group (55.7%, $n = 54$) at 3 months. Patients who had undergone DRG stimulation reported less paresthesia than the SCS group, with postural variation. At 12 months, 74.2% of the DRG arm achieved treatment success compared to 53.0% of the SCS group. These results suggest persistent effectiveness of DRG stimulation for CRPS patients. Patients from the DRG stimulation arm had significantly lower visual analogue scale scores throughout the 3-month period and continuing up to the 12-month endpoint of the study. In addition, patients who received DRG implantation continued the therapy for over 12 months without any issues in lead migration, contrary to that reported in patients who had undergone SCS.

A recent single-center study reported the promising effect of DRG stimulation for patients suffering from upper extremity CRPS.[3] After a DRG stimulation trial, 17 of 20 patients (85%) had 50% or greater improvement in pain scale ratings and underwent a permanent pulse generator implant, with all patients reporting 50% or greater pain relief at 6 months. Mean numeric rating scale (NRS) pain scores before DRG stimulation were 9.3 ± 1.1, with a mean reduction of 5.5 (95% confidence interval [CI], 4.5–6.6;p<0.001) at 6 months. Ten patients were taking opioids at baseline; the median (interquartile range) dose was 45 mg morphine equivalents (MME), which was reduced to 20 MME at 6 months. Of 17 patients with implants, 13 (76%) had continued 50% or greater improvement in NRS pain at 12 months. The median MME was slightly higher (25 MME) at 12 months. All patients with baseline MME of greater than 100 were reduced to regimens of less than 100 MME at 12 months with two patients completely weaned off their opioid use.[4]

PROS AND CONS OF DORSAL ROOT GANGLION STIMULATION

Like any medical intervention, DRG stimulation has its advantages and disadvantages for CRPS.[1,5]

Pros

- *Targeted pain relief.* DRG stimulation allows for precise targeting of pain signals at the source, which is particularly beneficial for patients with CRPS where pain can be localized to specific regions of the body. The cerebrospinal fluid layer surrounding the DRG has much lower volume than the one that surrounds the spinal cord. Therefore, lower stimulation amplitudes are required with DRG stimulation compared with SCS, resulting in less postural variation.

- *Selective stimulation*: DRG stimulation can provide pain relief without causing paresthesia (tingling sensation), making it a suitable option for patients who find paresthesia uncomfortable or unpleasant.
- *Pain reduction*: Studies have reported significant pain reduction and improved quality of life in CRPS patients who underwent DRG stimulation therapy.
- *Adjustability*: The therapy can be customized to individual patient needs, allowing for adjustments to stimulation parameters as pain patterns change.

Cons

- *Cost*: The initial cost of the device implantation and follow-up care can be high. DRG stimulation may not be widely available at all medical centers, thus limiting access for some patients.
- *Patient selection*: Not all CRPS patients are suitable candidates for DRG stimulation. Patient selection criteria are essential to identify those who are most likely to benefit from the therapy.
- *Long-term efficacy*: While DRG stimulation has shown promising results in clinical studies, the long-term effectiveness and durability of pain relief need further investigation.
- *Learning curve*: There might be a longer learning curve using DRG stimulation than SCS due to anatomical challenges in leads placement.

COMPLICATIONS OF DORSAL ROOT GANGLION STIMULATION

Most of the complications for DRG stimulation reported in the literature stem from device-related issues (47%) such as lead migration, lead damage, sheath damage, and erosion.[6] Among device-related complications, migration and lead damage were the most common, being reported 272 and 99 times out of 979 implants, respectively. Other complications related to the DRG procedure (28%), such as dura puncture, infection, and hematoma, were also reported. Though dural puncture is common with SCS, it is reported more frequently with DRG stimulation due to the complex manipulation required to insert the lead, sheath, and guidewires. Serious adverse events (SAEs) occurred in about 2.4% of cases. Literature also reported infection commonly associated with explants and revisions. Increased incidence of infection can be expected due to the increased length of time needed for implantation of the DRG stimulation device or the increased number of components in the system compared to those of SCS. No neurological deficits were reported, and the overall difference in SAEs between DRG stimulation and SCS was not clinically or statistically different.

CASE CONTINUATION

After a discussion of the options, efficacy, and pros and cons of neuromodulation, the patient elected to receive DRG stimulation, which provided him greater than 60% pain reduction. He was also able to reduce his oral analgesic intake and gradually increase motor activities with his foot and ankle.

KEY POINTS TO REMEMBER

- Dorsal root ganglion (DRG) stimulation has emerged as a novel neuromodulation modality for chronic complex regional pain syndrome (CRPS) pain in the lower extremity.
- DRG stimulation provides higher patient responder rate and less paresthesia compared to traditional SCS.
- The safety profile of DRG stimulation is comparable to traditional SCS.

Suggested Reading

Deer TR, Levy RM, Kramer J, et al. Dorsal root ganglion stimulation yielded higher treatment success rate for complex regional pain syndrome and causalgia at 3 and 12 months: A randomized comparative trial. *Pain*. 2017;158(4):669–681. doi:10.1097/j.pain.0000000000000814

Deer TR, Pope JE, Lamer TJ, et al. The Neuromodulation Appropriateness
Consensus Committee on best practices for dorsal root ganglion stimulation.
Neuromodulation. 2019;22(1):1–35. doi:10.1111/ner.12845

References

1. Deer TR, Pope JE, Lamer TJ, Grider JS, Provenzano D, Lubenow TR, et al. The
   Neuromodulation Appropriateness Consensus Committee on best practices for
   dorsal root ganglion stimulation. *Neuromodulation.* 2019;22:1–35.
2. Deer TR, Levy RM, Kramer J, Poree L, Amirdelfan K, Grigsby E, et al. Dorsal root
   ganglion stimulation yielded higher treatment success rate for complex regional
   pain syndrome and causalgia at 3 and 12 months: A randomized comparative
   trial. *Pain.* 2017;158:669–681.
3. Graca MJ, Lubenow TR, Landphair WR, Mccarthy RJ. Efficacy and safety
   of cervical and high-thoracic dorsal root ganglion stimulation therapy for
   complex regional pain syndrome of the upper extremities. *Neuromodulation.*
   2023;26:1781–1787.
4. Graca MJ, Lubenow TR. 2023. Update to "Efficacy and safety of cervical and
   high-thoracic dorsal root ganglion stimulation therapy for complex regional pain
   syndrome of the upper extremities." *Neuromodulation.* 2023;27(3):593–595.
5. Huygen F, Kallewaard JW, Nijhuis H, Liem L, Vesper J, Fahey ME, et al.
   Effectiveness and safety of dorsal root ganglion stimulation for the treatment of
   chronic pain: A pooled analysis. *Neuromodulation.* 2020;23:213–221.
6. Sivanesan E, Bicket MC, Cohen SP. Retrospective analysis of complications
   associated with dorsal root ganglion stimulation for pain relief in the FDA
   MAUDE database. *Reg Anesth Pain Med.* 2019;44:100–106.

It's Not All Central

Mark A. Chmiela and
Richard W. Rosenquist

Case

A 60-year-old woman presents for consultation with complaints of worsening severe left shoulder and proximal arm pain after undergoing arthroscopic rotator cuff repair 6 weeks ago. She reports restricted left shoulder range of motion; extreme pain across the shoulder and proximal arm to the level of the elbow, with associated swelling and redness; and an inability to wear a bra or tight shirt due to pain. She is unable to tolerate active or passive left shoulder abduction, and she exhibits allodynia over the shoulder and proximal arm. There is swelling, warmth, and erythema down to her elbow, but the forearm and hand are spared. She has failed conservative care, including physical therapy and multiple medications, and she recently underwent a subacromial bursa steroid injection with no relief. Her orthopedist informed her that there was no further surgical intervention appropriate for her. She reports significant pain affecting her quality of life and asks for your help.

What Do I Do Now?

TREATMENT-RESISTANT COMPLEX REGIONAL PAIN SYNDROME

Complex regional pain syndrome (CRPS) may develop after arthroscopic rotator cuff repair and pose a challenge for physicians to treat. While early intervention with physical and occupational therapy in conjunction with pharmacotherapy, biofeedback, and nerve blocks may provide relief in some patients, persistent neuropathic and sympathetically mediated pain may persist in many others, thus warranting further intervention.

NEUROMODULATION

Neuromodulation in the form of peripheral nerve stimulation (PNS) may provide meaningful relief in patients with CRPS of the extremities. In this case, the patient underwent an arthroscopic repair, which was followed by development of CRPS. Initially, a diagnostic suprascapular nerve block under fluoroscopic guidance provided approximately 60% relief of her symptoms for 1 week before her symptoms returned to baseline. A trial of PNS using two cylindrical leads placed percutaneously under fluoroscopic and ultrasound guidance targeting the suprascapular and axillary nerves was then pursued. Following a 1-week trial period, the patient reported greater than 70% relief of her pain symptoms in the shoulder and proximal arm with improvement in her range of motion. Permanent implantation was then performed with two leads placed percutaneously and anchored in place subcutaneously, allowing a radiofrequency transmitter to provide wireless stimulation to an implanted pulse generator (IPG). The patient continued to report meaningful relief of her symptoms. Alongside further physical therapy and medication management, the patient reported improved quality of life and functional ability.

DISEASE AND TREATMENT MECHANISMS

Although the pathophysiology of CRPS is not completely understood, evidence points to involvement of both the central and peripheral nervous systems. Damage to the peripheral nervous system due to trauma, whether accidental or as a result of surgery, can result in the induction of peripheral sensitization. This may be related to an increase in localized inflammatory mediators and a change in afferent nerve function leading to increases in spontaneous nociceptive activity. This, in turn, can result in central sensitization from sustained firing of afferent nociceptive A-Δ and C fibers. These can invoke changes within the dorsal horn and contribute to the development of persistent pain even when the noxious peripheral stimuli are removed.

In its current use, PNS is hypothesized to alter both the peripheral and central nervous systems. Within the periphery, nociceptive afferent transmission is mitigated by electrical activation of large diameter fibers causing nonpainful sensations. In addition, there may also be an effect on downregulating local inflammatory mediators at the site of injury within the periphery. At the level of the spinal cord, there is alteration of neurotransmitter activity, which results in an increase in inhibition of pain processing within the dorsal horn and a decrease in spinal cord inflammatory proteins. Through these actions and likely others, pain signaling is modulated in a way that results in decreased subjective pain perception in patients.

CANDIDATE SELECTION

PNS can be performed percutaneously for temporary treatment up to 60 days or implanted via a minimally invasive approach for permanent relief. Unlike spinal cord stimulation (SCS), PNS provides more focal targeting of injured nerves and is associated with decreased risks associated with neuraxial interventions. As CRPS has been known to spread to other areas and has been known to change characteristics with time, early intervention with neuromodulation after diagnosis may reduce further spread of CRPS and/or reduce the risk of chronic disease and functional limitations.

Although performed in this case, a diagnostic injection of the peripheral nerve is not required prior to pursuing a trial of neuromodulation. Success of PNS is independent of the response to a localized nerve block, which should not be considered as a decision point in the pursuit of neuromodulation. However, failure to respond meaningfully to a PNS trial of 5–7 days should tell the clinician that the patient is not an appropriate candidate for permanent implantation.

Clinicians are encouraged to consider PNS when an extremity is affected and where focal targeting of nerves innervating that area is possible.

Suggested Reading

Chmiela MA, Hendrickson M, Hale J, Liang C, Telefus P, Sagir A, Stanton-Hicks M. Direct peripheral nerve stimulation for the treatment of complex regional pain syndrome: A 30-year review. *Neuromodulation.* 2021;24(6):971–982. doi:10.1111/ner.13295

Deer TR, Eldabe S, Falowski SM, Huntoon MA, Staats PS, Cassar IR, et al. Peripherally induced reconditioning of the central nervous system: A proposed mechanistic theory for sustained relief of chronic pain with percutaneous peripheral nerve stimulation. *J Pain Res.* 2021;14:721–736. Published 2021 Mar 12. doi:10.2147/JPR.S297091

Fritz AV, Ferreira-Dos-Santos G, Hurdle MF, Clendenen S. Ultrasound-guided percutaneous peripheral nerve stimulation for the treatment of complex regional pain syndrome type 1 following a crush injury to the fifth digit: A rare case report. *Cureus.* 2019;11(12):e6506. Published 2019 Dec 29. doi:10.7759/cureus.6506

Helm S, Shirsat N, Calodney A, Abd-Elsayed A, Kloth D, Soin A, et al. Peripheral nerve stimulation for chronic pain: A systematic review of effectiveness and safety. Pain Ther. 2021;10(2):985–1002. doi:10.1007/s40122-021-00306-4

Lin T, Gargya A, Singh H, Sivanesan E, Gulati A. Mechanism of peripheral nerve stimulation in chronic pain. *Pain Med.* 2020;21(Suppl 1):S6–S12. doi:10.1093/pm/pnaa164

Perez RS, Zollinger PE, Dijkstra PU, Thomassen-Hilgersom IL, Zuurmond WW, Rosenbrand KC, et al. Evidence based guidelines for complex regional pain syndrome type 1. *BMC Neurol.* 2010;10:20. Published 2010 Mar 31. doi:10.1186/1471-2377-10-20

Poree L, Krames E, Pope J, Deer TR, Levy R, Schultz L. Spinal cord stimulation as treatment for complex regional pain syndrome should be considered earlier than last resort therapy. *Neuromodulation.* 2013;16(2):125–141. doi:10.1111/ner.12035

Visnjevac O, Costandi S, Patel BA, Azer G, Agarwal P, Bolash R, Mekhail NA. A comprehensive outcome-specific review of the use of spinal cord stimulation for complex regional pain syndrome. *Pain Pract.* 2017;17(4):533–545. doi:10.1111/papr.1251

9 Dissociative Experience

Alexander Foster, Magdalena Anitescu, Pavan Tankha, and Jijun Xu

Case

A 41-year-old woman without significant past medical
history had an injury to her right elbow and wrist
during an accident. After being taken to the emergency
room, she had an x-ray of the affected limb that did not
show acute abnormalities. The patient was diagnosed
with a contusion. Pain in the area began to increase
gradually, accompanied by new, non-pitting edema
of the right hand and forearm. Hyperesthesia also
developed to the point where even air blowing on the
affected limb caused her anxiety. This was followed
soon by hypertrichosis, as well as a palpable difference
in temperature between her right and left hands. Both
active and passive range of motion of the affected
limb were restricted. A diagnosis of complex regional
pain syndrome (CRPS) was made. The patient had
failed numerous pharmacological therapies, including
amitriptyline, gabapentin, opioids, and lidocaine cream.
The patient had read in medical news that intravenous
ketamine infusion is effective in managing CRPS pain.

What Do I Do Now?

OVERVIEW

Ketamine is a chemical derivative of the illicit drug phencyclidine (PCP). Its use as an anesthetic began in the 1960s. However, it was quickly abandoned as a sole agent due to demonstrated severe emergence delirium. As for its mechanism of action, it is thought to be involved in signaling at more than 10 distinct receptor pathways, resulting in a wide array of neurological, cardiovascular, and pulmonary effects.[1] The US Drug Enforcement Administration (DEA) has listed ketamine as a Schedule III controlled substance due to its low-to-moderate potential for abuse, psychological dependence, and physical dependence. Administration of ketamine should be strictly regulated by DEA, local, and state laws.

Intravenous ketamine infusion has been used to treat refractory chronic pain, including pain from complex regional pain syndrome (CRPS).[2-5] Two randomized controlled trials reported significant pain relief in patients with CRPS.[6,7] A consensus panel concluded that there is moderate evidence supporting intravenous ketamine infusion (22 mg/hr for 4 days or 0.35 mg/kg/hr over 4 hours daily for 10 days) for CRPS.[2,3,8,9]

Major contraindications for IV ketamine infusion include pregnancy, active psychosis, elevated intracranial or intraocular pressure, active substance abuse, severe liver disease, and poorly controlled cardiovascular disease.[2] Side effects of ketamine use include hypersalivation, dizziness, nausea and vomiting, tachycardia, hypertension, and palpation. Psychoactive symptoms, hepatic injury, and possible cystitis have limited its use.[1] A recent preclinical study indicated that ketamine is less addictive than cocaine thanks to its N-methyl-D-aspartic acid (NMDA) receptor antagonism.[10] However, tolerance to ketamine's antidepressant and antinociceptive effects have been reported.[11] Patients with CRPS receiving long-term (≥6 months) frequent (two times or more per month) ketamine treatment can develop impairment in cognitive function.[12]

PRE-INFUSION ASSESSMENT

Pre-infusion assessment should include a comprehensive history (to rule out contraindications shown above) and airway assessment. Per consensus guidelines,[2] no testing is recommended prior to ketamine infusion for healthy individuals. A baseline echocardiogram maybe considered to exclude uncontrolled ischemic heart disease. Baseline and post-infusion liver function tests should be considered if there are risk factors for liver toxicity.[2]

INFUSION PROTOCOL

Data on intravenous ketamine infusion for pediatric CRPS patients are lacking. The following consensus protocol is for adult patients with refractory CRPS.[13] Anesthesiology practice guidelines advise that those administering the infusion must be trained in conscious sedation, airway management, and advanced cardiac life support (ACLS).[14] The infusion can be conducted at either inpatient wards or outpatient clinics. The range of dose and duration can be determined by patient tolerability, response (i.e., pain relief) to the infusion, and logistic considerations. Adjuvant medications, including clonidine, midazolam, and ondansetron, can be administered to mitigate ketamine-induced cardiovascular, psychotic, and emetic effects, respectively. It is recommended that heart rate, blood pressure, pulse oximetry, and level of consciousness be monitored during infusion treatments. Patients at high risk of adverse respiratory events should also have their end-tidal carbon dioxide continuously monitored. During infusion(s), a Foley catheter or portable urinal should be used to monitor urine output for calculation of intake/output variance. Intermittent pneumatic compression devices should be applied to prevent deep venous thrombosis.[13]

Inpatient Continuous Infusion

Inpatient therapy should take place in an intensive care unit–type setting with full ACLS capability.[13]

Initial rate is 10 mg/hr (approximately 0.15 mg/kg/hr based on ideal body weight). This is increased every 2 hours in 5–10 mg increments. Titrate to "drowsy-to-moderate sedation" per the Richmond Agitation and Sedation Scale (RASS) score of –1 to –3 or pain reduction by 50% using a numeric pain rating scale. If the patient becomes oversedated or dissociation is not tolerated, then infusion may be reduced by 25%. The maximum rate is 25 mg/hr. The duration is 24 hours daily for 3–5 days. Tapering can be done at 10 mg/hr, if needed.

Outpatient Intermittent Infusion

Outpatient infusion should take place in a suite with continuous, direct cardiorespiratory monitoring and one-on-one or continuous remote audio-visual monitoring by trained medical personnel, at a minimum. Full ACLS capability must be maintained.

Initial rate on Day 1 is 0.2 mg/kg/hr for 4 hours, titrated every hour by 0.05 mg/kg/hr increments to a RASS score of –1 to –3, or pain reduction by 50% using a numerical pain rating scale. If the patient becomes oversedated or dissociation is not tolerated, then infusion may be reduced by 25%. The maximum rate is 50 mg/hr. The total maximum dose is 200 mg on Day 1. With subsequent sessions, dosing is 25–30% more than the prior day's maximum dose. The target dose is 75–125 mg/hr or 300–500 mg daily over 4 hours for a duration of 5–10 days. A recent study reported that 4 days of treatment are sufficient for CRPS in the lower extremity while longer duration of treatment might be needed for upper extremity CRPS pain.[15] No tapering is needed for intermittent infusions.

POST-INFUSION MANAGEMENT

Post-infusion monitoring should continue for 6 hours after inpatient therapy and 60 minutes after outpatient therapy. Inpatients require a sitter/minder for 3 days and daily serum liver panels for 3 days. Outpatients require a (nonprofessional) sitter/minder through the first night.[13]

Patient should be followed up at 2–3 months after the infusion. Thirty percent or greater pain relief lasting over 3 weeks in conjunction with patient satisfaction is considered a positive outcome.[2] A recent study reported that patients who had a positive response to sympathetic nerve block and patients who were obese were more likely to respond positively to ketamine infusion.[16] Subsequent ("booster") infusion can be considered based on patient's tolerability and response to the infusion. Inpatient booster sessions are considered optional, with a starting dose of 25% of the maximum dose during the previous inpatient therapy. For outpatients, the 5- to 10-day infusion session can be repeated after 3–6 months.

FUTURE DIRECTIONS

Overall, the current level of evidence in ketamine infusion for CRPS is moderate at best. Future studies with greater power (e.g., double-blinded, randomized, placebo-controlled trials) are warranted to guide the use of this treatment modality for CRPS. A true placebo for ketamine infusion is yet to be identified.

KEY POINTS TO REMEMBER

- There is moderate evidence supporting intravenous ketamine infusion (22 mg/hr for 4 days or 0.35 mg/kg/hr over 4 hours daily for 10 days) for chronic pain in complex regional pain syndrome (CRPS).
- Patients who are obese and who have had positive responses to sympathetic blocks might be more likely to respond to ketamine infusion.
- Long-term frequent use of ketamine may lead to tolerance, addiction, and cognitive impairments.

Suggested Reading

Cohen SP, Bhatia A, Buvanendran A, Schwenk ES, Wasan AD, Hurley RW, et al. Consensus guidelines on the use of intravenous ketamine infusions for chronic pain from the American Society of Regional Anesthesia and Pain Medicine, the American Academy of Pain Medicine, and the American Society of Anesthesiologists. *Reg Anesth Pain Med*. 2018;43:521–546.

Schwartzman RJ, Alexander GM, Grothusen JR, Paylor T, Reichenberger E, Perreault M. Outpatient intravenous ketamine for the treatment of complex regional pain syndrome: A double-blind placebo controlled study. *Pain*. 2009;147:107–115.

Sigtermans MJ, Van Hilten JJ, Bauer MC, Arbous MS, Marinus J, Sarton EY, Dahan A. Ketamine produces effective and long-term pain relief in patients with complex regional pain syndrome type 1. *Pain*. 2009;145:304–311.

References

1. Li L, Vlisides PE. Ketamine: 50 years of modulating the mind. *Front Hum Neurosci*. 2016;10:612.

2. Cohen SP, Bhatia A, Buvanendran A, Schwenk ES, Wasan AD, Hurley RW, et al. Consensus guidelines on the use of intravenous ketamine infusions for chronic pain from the American Society of Regional Anesthesia and Pain Medicine, the American Academy of Pain Medicine, and the American Society of Anesthesiologists. *Reg Anesth Pain Med*. 2018;43:521–546.

3. Orhurhu V, Orhurhu MS, Bhatia A, Cohen SP. Ketamine infusions for chronic pain: A systematic review and meta-analysis of randomized controlled trials. *Anesth Analg*. 2019;129:241–254.

4. Patil S, Anitescu M. Efficacy of outpatient ketamine infusions in refractory chronic pain syndromes: A 5-year retrospective analysis. *Pain Med*. 2021;13:263–269.

5. Mangnus TJP, Dirckx M, Bharwani KD, De Vos CC, Frankema SPG, Stronks DL, Huygen F. Effect of intravenous low-dose S-ketamine on pain in patients with complex regional pain syndrome: A retrospective cohort study. *Pain Pract*. 2021;21:890–897.

6. Sigtermans MJ, Van Hilten JJ, Bauer MC, Arbous MS, Marinus, J, Sarton EY, Dahan A. Ketamine produces effective and long-term pain relief in patients with complex regional pain syndrome type 1. *Pain*. 2009;145:304–311.

7. Schwartzman RJ, Alexander GM, Grothusen JR, Paylor, T, Reichenberger E, Perreault M. Outpatient intravenous ketamine for the treatment of complex regional pain syndrome: A double-blind placebo controlled study. *Pain*. 2009;147:107–115.

8. Xu J, Yang J, Lin P, Rosenquist E, Cheng J. Intravenous therapies for complex regional pain syndrome: A systematic review. *Anesth Analg*. 2016;122:843–856.

9. Zhao J, Wang Y, Wang D. The effect of ketamine infusion in the treatment of complex regional pain syndrome: A systemic review and meta-analysis. *Curr Pain Headache Rep*. 2018;22:12.

10. Simmler LD, Li Y, Hadjas LC, Hiver A, Van Zessen R, Luscher C. Dual action of ketamine confines addiction liability. *Nature*. 2022;608:368–373.

11. Bonnet U. Long-term ketamine self-injections in major depressive disorder: Focus on tolerance in ketamine's antidepressant response and the development of ketamine addiction. *J Psychoactive Drugs*. 2015;47:276–285.

12. Kim M, Cho S, Lee JH. The effects of long-term ketamine treatment on cognitive function in complex regional pain syndrome: A preliminary study. *Pain Med*. 2016;17:1447–1451.

13. Xu J, Herndon C, Anderson S, Getson P, Foorsov V, Harbut RE, et al. Intravenous ketamine infusion for complex regional pain syndrome: Survey, consensus, and a reference protocol. *Pain Med*. 2019;20:323–334.

14. American Society of Anesthesiologists Task Force on Chronic Pain Management, American Society of Regional Anesthesia and Pain Medicine. Practice

guidelines for chronic pain management: An updated report by the American Society of Anesthesiologists Task Force on Chronic Pain Management and the American Society of Regional Anesthesia and Pain Medicine. *Anesthesiology*. 2010;112:810–833.

15. Kirkpatrick AF, Saghafi A, Yang K, Qiu P, Alexander J, Bavry E, Schwartzman R. Optimizing the treatment of CRPS with ketamine. *Clin J Pain*. 2020;36:516–523.

16. Cohen SP, Khunsriraksakul C, Yoo Y, Parker E, Samen-Akinsiku CDK, Patel N, et al. Sympathetic blocks as a predictor for response to ketamine infusion in patients with complex regional pain syndrome: A multicenter study. *Pain Med*. 2023;24:316–324.

10 Migration and Capture

Jagan Devarajan and Beth Minzter

Case

A 40-year-old woman is referred to the pain clinic
with painful swelling of her right hand and right
and left legs. She experienced trauma to her right
hand 18 months ago and was diagnosed with a
scaphoid bone fracture, treated conservatively with
immobilization for 4 weeks. Right hand pain gradually
worsened in severity and subsequently spread to the
right upper and lower extremity with accompanying
altered sensation, severe cold intolerance, and muscle
weakness. Her right leg was swollen and tender with
cold and sweaty skin. Right lower extremity also
exhibited hyperalgesia, allodynia, and edema with
no sensorimotor dysfunction. Four weeks later, she
developed painful swelling with sudomotor changes
in her left leg as well. The patient is frustrated about
the spread of the pain from the initial trauma area and
wants to know why and how to manage it.

What Do I Do Now?

SPREAD OF COMPLEX REGIONAL PAIN SYNDROME FROM ITS ORIGINAL BODY SITE TO A DISTANT SITE

Complex regional pain syndrome (CRPS) usually starts in one limb and can spread to other places. This is probably one of, if not the most, concerning issues associated with CRPS. The spread of CRPS has been reported as early as 1976, when Kozin et al. reported 11 cases of spread with bilateral involvement.[1] The patients in these cases responded well to corticosteroids. Abnormal results were identified via both quantitative clinical methods and synovial biopsy and confirmed bilateral spread of the disease. The incidence of spread or bilateral or multiple involvement of CRPS is 48%.[2] The exact pathogenesis is not known, however the theories of genetic predisposition, aberrant regulation of neurogenic inflammation, and maladaptive neuronal plasticity are proposed to result in spread of CRPS. Rommel et al. proposed a supraspinal mechanism.[3] He proposed functional alterations in the thalamus, which relays sensory information and changes associated with CRPS across the hemisphere, to explain contralateral spread. Spinal and thalamic mechanisms underlie contralateral spread, and cortical mechanisms underpin spontaneous spread in an ipsilateral pattern. Rarely do systemic factors result in spread to unusual areas, such as the eye or abdomen, for example.

CRPS can occasionally spread beyond the extremities as well. In addition, it can evolve into a full-blown fibromyalgia picture. The phenotypic changes in dorsal root ganglia (DRG) and small-fiber neuropathy are responsible for linking the painful disorders of CRPS with fibromyalgia.[4]

SPREAD PATTERN OF CRPS

Five different types of patterns of spread are reported in the literature.

- *Contiguous spread*: CRPS spreads within the affected extremity and usually presents with gradual enlargement of the affected area, from distal to proximal, and then moves up the limb or body proximally.
- *Contralateral or "mirror image" spread*: Symptoms and signs appear on the opposite side of the body in an area closely matching the location of the area originally affected.

- *Independent spread*: New symptoms or signs appear in an area distant to, independent of, and noncontiguous with the area originally affected.
- *Ipsilateral spread*: CRPS spreads to either the upper or lower extremity or the face on the same side of the body as the area originally affected.
- *Diagonal spread*: This is a rare type of spread associated with the appearance of symptoms in the limb diagonally opposite to the one originally affected.

In patients with CRPS in multiple limbs, spontaneous spread of symptoms generally follows a contralateral (49%) or ipsilateral pattern (30%), whereas diagonal spread (14%) is rare and generally preceded by a new trauma.[5]

PREDISPOSING FACTORS ASSOCIATED WITH SPREAD OF CRPS

Younger age of onset and severe initial signs and symptoms are associated with a significantly higher risk of spread of CRPS.[6] Patients with movement disorders have a higher risk of spread of the disease. The hazard of spread of CRPS increases with the number of limbs affected. The other putative risk factors for spread are female gender, greater duration of the disease, and preceding soft tissue trauma or surgery or any intervention.[7]

TYPICAL CHARACTERISTICS OF SPREAD

The median interval between the appearance of symptoms in one limb and that in the other limb is 21 months ($n = 24$, range 2–95) for contralateral spread, whereas the interval was 19 months ($n = 13$, range 3–58) for ipsilateral spread and 10 months ($n = 1$) for diagonal spread. There are no statistically significant differences between ipsilateral and contralateral spread of the disease. Compared to risk of contralateral spread (hazard reference ratio of 1.0), the hazard ratio associated with ipsilateral spread was 0.44 (95% confidence interval [CI]: 0.22–0.89) and that of diagonal spread is 0.04 (CI: 0.005–0.30). Presence of CRPS in additional limbs significantly increases the risk of developing CRPS in subsequent limbs. The characteristics and pattern of development of CRPS symptoms and signs after new trauma are different from that of CRPS that spreads without new trauma.[8,9]

PATHOGENIC MECHANISMS OF DIFFERENT PATTERNS OF CRPS SPREAD

The underlying pathogenesis of ipsilateral spread and contralateral spread is different from that of spread with and without new trauma. Spontaneous spread to the contralateral limb was 2.3 times more likely than spread to the ipsilateral limb and 25 times more likely than diagonal spread. The fact that CRPS spread more commonly in younger patients and that their siblings are at higher risk of developing CRPS indicates that genetic factors are likely to play a role in the development of chronicity and spread of CRPS.[6] Different human leukocyte antigen class I and II factors have been associated with spread of CRPS.

Cortical and spinal-mediated mechanisms play a more dominant role in the spread of CRPS than do systemic predisposing factors. The pathogenesis of contralateral spread is largely unknown; however, it is becoming increasingly evident from both human and animal studies that altered spinal processing of incoming information is responsible for the development of neuropathic symptoms in the opposite side of the body. The aberrant sensory information is carried by growth factors secreted by commissural interneurons in spinal and brainstem neurons. In addition to growth factors, proinflammatory cytokines and spinal glia cells have also been shown to play a role in the development of contralateral symptoms.[10–12] Moreover, whole-head magneto-encephalography has demonstrated that unilateral tactile stimuli in patients with CRPS can cause abnormal bilateral activation in both primary somatosensory cortices. This may explain bilateral or contralateral spread. In a case report by Buntjen et al., pain distribution as a result of CRPS matches abnormal cortical sensory misrepresentation. Hence the authors suggest that cortical reorganization processes may be responsible for the development and spread of CRPS.[13] However, Mancini et al. refuted the cortical reorganization process associated with CRPS.[14] Koltsenburg et al. identified DRG changes associated with any nerve injury.[8] They demonstrated four different histopathological changes in the DRG of the same segment in response to a nerve injury on the opposite side.

In contrast, spinal cord–mediated changes are mainly responsible for the development of axial or ipsilateral symptoms of CRPS. Similar to many neurological disorders such as amyotrophic lateral sclerosis and polio, glial-mediated changes in one segment of the spinal cord can spread to remote segments by axonal transport via descending or ascending fiber tracts.[15] Del Valle et al. reported a significant loss of posterior horn cells and activation of both microglia and astrocytes at the initial site of injury as well as throughout the entire length of the spinal cord in patients with CRPS.[16] This supports the hypothesis that the segmental changes induced by CRPS in the spinal cord are not restricted to a dermatomal or myotomal pattern and instead extend rostrally and caudally from the initially affected segmental regions. Rommel et al. also proposed that functional alterations in the thalamus are responsible for the entire hemisensory impairment in patients with CRPS that affects one extremity.[3]

In general, supraspinal glia and glial-derived proinflammatory cytokines may play a major role in spread of CRPS, just as they do for any pain modulation.

MANAGEMENT OF CRPS SPREAD

CRPS spread is considered a late stage of the disease. It is complex and follows a debilitating course. At this later stage, CRPS is difficult to treat and often refractory to conventional interventional and management modalities. Treatment should be multidisciplinary and multipronged. All patients should be offered physical and occupational therapy which incorporates mobilization, mirror therapy, and desensitization. Acupuncture, treatment of psychological comorbidities, and biofeedback may be considered as well.

Pharmacological management such as steroids, antidepressants, anticonvulsants, bisphosphonates, and calcium can be tried per institutional protocol.[17,18] Ketamine and cannabinoids may also be included in the treatment armamentarium.

Routine management protocol for CRPS should be followed for individual organs or body parts. For example, upper and lower extremity CRPS should be managed by conservative therapy followed by either stellate ganglion or lumbar plexus block, respectively. If chemical sympathectomy provides temporary relief, radiofrequency ablation, surgical, or chemical (neurolytic) destructive options may be considered. Clinicians must be cognizant, however, of one review that reports that sympathectomized patients were at higher risk of spread of CRPS (37% of patients) in contrast to 18% of the remaining patients who had not undergone sympathectomy.

Unless there is an underlying abnormality in nerve conduction or tissues, surgery should be avoided at all costs.[19] Surgery can act as a precipitating factor for the spread of the disease and can result in its rapid progression. This further adds neuropathic pain to the differential diagnosis. Cherington et al. showed that unnecessary or unsuccessful surgery is the strongest predictor of spread of CRPS and poor treatment outcome.[19]

Neuromodulation is increasingly being utilized in the treatment of CRPS. There is a diverse range of neuromodulatory treatment options available. Transcutaneous nerve stimulation is the least invasive of these. Spinal cord stimulation is commonly used.[20,21] Other options include peripheral nerve stimulation,[22] DRG stimulation,[23] noninvasive brain stimulation,[24] and deep brain stimulation.[25]

KEY POINTS TO REMEMBER

- The spread of complex regional pain syndrome (CRPS) can occur in later stages of the disease and can affect different regions of the body, with contralateral spread the most common occurrence.
- The underlying mechanisms of spread are attributed to cortical reorganization and spinal-mediated changes.
- Supraspinal glia and glial-derived proinflammatory cytokines can accelerate the spread of the disease, making anti-inflammatory measures a common prevention method.

- Several theories have been proposed to explain this phenomenon. In addition to genetic predisposition, aberrant regulation of neurogenic inflammation and maladaptive neuronal plasticity have also been proposed. Despite these theories, more research is needed to fully understand the underlying pathogenesis of CRPS spread.
- Due to its resistance to common management strategies, early diagnosis and aggressive control of the primary disease is crucial to prevent the development and spread of CRPS.

Suggested Reading

Maleki J, LeBel AA, Bennett GJ, Schwartzman RJ. Patterns of spread in complex regional pain syndrome, type I (reflex sympathetic dystrophy). *Pain*. 2000 Dec 1;88(3):259–266.

van Rijn MA, Marinus J, Putter H, Bosselaar SRJ, Moseley GL, van Hilten JJ. Spreading of complex regional pain syndrome: Not a random process. *J Neural Transm*. 2011 Sep;118(9):1301–1309.

Watkins LR, Maier SF. Beyond neurons: Evidence that immune and glial cells contribute to pathological pain states. *Physiol Rev*. 2002 Oct;82(4):981–1011.

References

1. Kozin F, McCarty DJ, Sims J, Genant H. The reflex sympathetic dystrophy syndrome. I. Clinical and histologic studies: Evidence for bilaterality, response to corticosteroids and articular involvement. *Am J Med*. 1976 Mar;60(3):321–331.

2. van Rijn MA, Marinus J, Putter H, Bosselaar SRJ, Moseley GL, van Hilten JJ. Spreading of complex regional pain syndrome: Not a random process. *J Neural Transm*. 2011 Sep;118(9):1301–1309.

3. Rommel O, Gehling M, Dertwinkel R, Witscher K, Zenz M, Malin JP, et al. Hemisensory impairment in patients with complex regional pain syndrome. *Pain*. 1999 Mar;80(1–2):95–101.

4. Martínez-Lavín M, Vargas A, Silveira LH, Amezcua-Guerra LM, MartíMartnez-Laviínez-Martínez L-A, Pineda C. Complex regional pain syndrome evolving to full-blown fibromyalgia: A proposal of common mechanisms. *J Clin Rheumatol*. 2021 Sep 1;27(6S):S274–S277.

5. Maleki J, LeBel AA, Bennett GJ, Schwartzman RJ. Patterns of spread in complex regional pain syndrome, type I (reflex sympathetic dystrophy). *Pain*. 2000 Dec 1;88(3):259–266.

6. de Rooij AM, de Mos M, van Hilten JJ, Sturkenboom MCJM, Gosso MF, van den Maagdenberg AMJM, et al. Increased risk of complex regional pain syndrome in siblings of patients? *J Pain*. 2009 Dec;10(12):1250–1255.

7. Modarresi S, Aref-Eshghi E, Walton DM, MacDermid JC. Does a familial subtype of complex regional pain syndrome exist? Results of a systematic review. *Can J Pain*. 2019 Jan 1;3(1):157–166.

8. Koltzenburg M, Wall PD, McMahon SB. Does the right side know what the left is doing? *Trends Neurosci*. 1999 Mar;22(3):122–127.

9. Hatashita S, Sekiguchi M, Kobayashi H, Konno S, Kikuchi S. Contralateral neuropathic pain and neuropathology in dorsal root ganglion and spinal cord following hemilateral nerve injury in rats. *Spine*. 2008 May 20;33(12):1344–1351.

10. Watkins LR, Maier SF. Beyond neurons: Evidence that immune and glial cells contribute to pathological pain states. *Physiol Rev*. 2002 Oct;82(4):981–1011.

11. Milligan ED, Twining C, Chacur M, Biedenkapp J, O'Connor K, Poole S, et al. Spinal glia and proinflammatory cytokines mediate mirror-image neuropathic pain in rats. *J Neurosci*. 2003 Feb 1;23(3):1026–1040.

12. Iwatsuki K, Hoshiyama M, Yoshida A, Uemura J-I, Hoshino A, Morikawa I, et al. Chronic pain-related cortical neural activity in patients with complex regional pain syndrome. *IBRO Neuroscience Reports*. 2021 Jun;10:208–215.

13. Büntjen L, Hopf J-M, Merkel C, Voges J, Knape S, Heinze H-J, et al. Somatosensory misrepresentation associated with chronic pain: Spatiotemporal correlates of sensory perception in a patient following a complex regional pain syndrome spread. *Front Neurol*. 2017 Apr 10;8:142.

14. Mancini F, Wang AP, Schira MM, Isherwood ZJ, McAuley JH, Iannetti GD, et al. Fine-grained mapping of cortical somatotopies in chronic complex regional pain syndrome. *J Neurosci*. 2019 Nov 13;39(46):9185–9196.

15. Brooks BR. The role of axonal transport in neurodegenerative disease spread: A meta-analysis of experimental and clinical poliomyelitis compares with amyotrophic lateral sclerosis. *Can J Neurol Sci*. 1991 Aug;18(3 Suppl):435–438.

16. Del Valle L, Schwartzman RJ, Alexander G. Spinal cord histopathological alterations in a patient with longstanding complex regional pain syndrome. *Brain Behav Immun*. 2009 Jan;23(1):85–91.

17. Jamroz A, Berger M, Winston P. Prednisone for acute complex regional pain syndrome: A retrospective cohort study. *Pain Res Manag*. 2020 Feb 25;2020:8182569.

18. Kleiber B, Jain S, Trivedi MH. Depression and pain: Implications for symptomatic presentation and pharmacological treatments. *Psychiatry (Edgmont)*. 2005 May;2(5):12–18. www.rsdrx.com/CRPS_824_Patients_Article.pdf

19. Cherington M, Happer I, Machanic B, Parry L. Surgery for thoracic outlet syndrome may be hazardous to your health. *Muscle Nerve*. 1986 Sep;9(7):632–634.

20. Martini ML, Caridi JM, Zeldin L, Neifert SN, Nistal DA, Kim JD, et al. Perioperative outcomes of spinal cord stimulator placement in patients with complex regional pain syndrome compared with patients without complex regional pain syndrome. *World Neurosurg*. 2020 May;137:e106–e117.
21. Risson EG, Serpa AP, Berger JJ, Koerbel RFH, Koerbel A. Spinal cord stimulation in the treatment of complex regional pain syndrome type 1: Is trial truly required? *Clin Neurol Neurosurg*. 2018 Aug;171:156–162.
22. Chmiela MA, Hendrickson M, Hale J, Liang C, Telefus P, Sagir A, et al. Direct peripheral nerve stimulation for the treatment of complex regional pain syndrome: A 30-year review. *Neuromodulation*. 2021 Aug;24(6):971–982.
23. Ghosh P, Gungor S. Utilization of concurrent dorsal root ganglion stimulation and dorsal column spinal cord stimulation in complex regional pain syndrome. *Neuromodulation*. 2021 Jun;24(4):769–773.
24. O'Connell NE, Wand BM, Marston L, Spencer S, Desouza LH. Non-invasive brain stimulation techniques for chronic pain. *Cochrane Database Syst Rev*. 2014 Apr 11;(4):CD008208.
25. Galafassi GZ, Simm Pires de Aguiar PH, Simm RF, Franceschini PR, Filho MP, Pagura JR, et al. Neuromodulation for medically refractory neuropathic pain: Spinal cord stimulation, deep brain stimulation, motor cortex stimulation, and posterior insula stimulation. *World Neurosurg*. 2021 Feb;146:246–260.

How to Avoid a Nightmare

Zhuo Sun, Wenbao Wang,
and Shiqian Shen

Case

A 64-year-old woman presented to the emergency
department with a distal radius fracture after falling
from a ladder. Her medical history included complex
regional pain syndrome (CRPS) on her right ankle
resulting from ankle surgery and fibromyalgia. An
x-ray revealed that her fracture was unstable, and
the orthopedic surgeon planned to perform internal
fixation surgery. The patient, whose current numerical
rating scale pain score was 10/10, was otherwise
stable. She voiced deep concern about developing
CRPS after surgery and asked if anything could be
done to prevent it.

What Do I Do Now?

WHAT IS KNOWN ABOUT PREVENTION OF CRPS?

Complex regional pain syndrome (CRPS) is a debilitating pain condition with unclear etiology, although it has been associated with surgery or trauma. With limited treatment options and often poor outcomes, prevention of CRPS is of utmost importance, especially for high-risk patients.

Risk factors related to CRPS are multifactorial and include age over 60 years, female gender, existing fibromyalgia, fracture of long bones, a high number of manipulations, comorbidities, and a previous history of CRPS (Louis et al., 2023, Taylor et al., 2021). In addition to patient-related factors, treatment modality has also been investigated as a possible risk factor. Surgery itself, including a variety of upper extremity surgeries, has been associated with the development of CRPS.

CRPS is not an uncommon surgical complication. Optimizing perioperative treatment such as pharmacological and regional analgesic techniques may aid in the prevention of postsurgical CRPS. The optimal timing for surgery in patients at high risk for CRPS remains unknown. Some practitioners prefer to wait until the signs and symptoms of CRPS (e.g., edema, temperature asymmetry, skin color changes of the affected limb) have abated (Harden et al., 2003, Marx et al., 2001). For elective surgeries, some recommend the use of peripheral vasodilators or sympathetic nervous system blockade to increase blood flow until skin temperature is normal. Others recommend that elective surgeries be delayed until CRPS symptoms are under good control after a series of sympathetic blocks.

In addition to sympathetic blocks, intravenous regional blocks with lidocaine and clonidine have demonstrated benefits in the perioperative treatment of patients with CRPS in prospective, randomized controlled clinical trials. Preoperative use of brachial plexus block also has been suggested to prevent CRPS in upper extremity surgery. A recent study demonstrated that adding 500 mg of vitamin C to the local anesthetic in a Bier block significantly reduces the incidence of CRPS after distal radius fractures. Some case reports have shown that epidural analgesia injection can reduce the incidence of postoperative CRPS.

Preoperative pain has been shown to be a predictor of CRPS through altered central nociceptive processing pathways. Harden et al. reported that patients with increased preoperative pain had a higher chance of developing postoperative CRPS after total knee arthroplasty (Harden et al., 2003).

Commenting on this finding, the authors noted that it is imperative to thoroughly assess and properly manage pain before surgery.

There is evidence that *preventative analgesic techniques*, which aim to reduce central hyperexcitability, demonstrate analgesic benefit and are likely to prevent postsurgical CRPS. Because it is difficult to achieve total or optimal pain relief with a single drug or method, multimodal analgesic techniques have been applied perioperatively (Perez et al., 2010). In a retrospective study of 1,200 patients undergoing anterior cruciate ligament (ACL) surgery, a standard postoperative analgesic group was compared to a preemptive multimodal group, which received an extra dose of 1,000 mg acetaminophen every 6 hours and 50 mg rofecoxib daily starting 48 hours before surgery. In addition, a femoral nerve block and an intraarticular injection of bupivacaine-clonidine-morphine were performed 30 minutes before surgery. There was a significantly lower incidence of CRPS in the preemptive multimodal group (4%) compared to the standard care group (1%) at 1-year follow-up. In addition to providing significant postoperative analgesia after arthroscopic knee surgery, intravenous regional block with clonidine has also been shown to be effective in managing CRPS of the knee.

A variety of drugs have been administered perioperatively to decrease the incidence of CRPS after surgical procedures, among them are calcitonin, carnitine, corticosteroids, ketanserin, vitamin C, and mannitol. Of those pharmacologic agents, only vitamin C has been shown to be beneficial in prophylactic treatment of CRPS in prospective, placebo-controlled studies. One recent meta-analysis found that vitamin C (500 mg/d for 50 days) may halve the risk of CRPS within the first year after a distal radius fracture. However, because of the limited number of high-level studies, the American Academy of Orthopedic Surgeons Clinical Practice Guidelines on Distal Radius Fractures recently downgraded the recommendation of adjuvant vitamin C in CRPS prophylaxis to moderate. Since the risk related to taking vitamin C is extremely low, perioperative vitamin C administration could be considered as a modality of CRPS prophylaxis for high-risk patients.

Postoperative physical therapy is always recommended after orthopedic surgical procedures. Patients who are unable to participate in a rehabilitation program after arthroscopic knee surgery may be at increased risk for CRPS. Prospective, randomized, controlled clinical trials have demonstrated the efficacy of physical therapy in reducing pain and improving active mobility in patients with CRPS. Postoperative physical therapy and rehabilitation in conjunction with preemptive multimodal techniques seems promising, but further research is needed.

A PRACTICAL PREVENTION PLAN

The case patient's concern was addressed with the following recommendations:

- Achieve significant pain relief before going into surgery.
- Initiate perioperative vitamin C.
- Perform preoperative brachial plexus block.
- Apply preemptive multimodal technique with use of acetaminophen and rofecoxib.
- Start physical therapy and rehabilitation after surgery.

KEY POINTS TO REMEMBER

- Postoperative complex regional pain syndrome (CRPS) after orthopedic surgery is not uncommon, and prevention is recommended, especially for high-risk patients.
- Elective surgeries should be delayed until CRPS symptoms are under control.
- Perioperative optimization with pharmacologic and regional analgesic techniques may prevent the development of CRPS after surgery.
- Multimodal analgesic techniques ought to be applied perioperatively.
- Perioperative sympathectomy, with or without general anesthesia, may be advantageous for CRPS patients who require surgery.
- Vitamin C has been shown to be beneficial in the prophylactic treatment of CRPS in prospective, placebo-controlled studies.
- Postoperative physical therapy and rehabilitation in conjunction with preemptive multimodal techniques seems promising, but further research is needed.

Suggested Reading

Harden NR, Bruehl S, Stanos S, Brander V, Chung OY, Saltz S, Adams A, Stulberg DS. Prospective examination of pain-related and psychological predictors of CRPS-like phenomena following total knee arthroplasty: A preliminary study. *Pain.* 2003;106:393–400.

Louis MH, Meyer C, Legrain V, Berquin A. Biological and psychological early prognostic factors in complex regional pain syndrome: A systematic review. *Eur J Pain.* 2023;27:338–352.

Marx C, Wiedersheim P, Michel BA, Stucki G. Preventing recurrence of reflex sympathetic dystrophy in patients requiring an operative intervention at the site of dystrophy after surgery. *Clin Rheumatol.* 2021;20:114–118.

Perez RS, Zollinger PE, Dijkstra PU, Thomassen-Hilgersom IL, Zuurmond WW, Rosenbrand KC, et al. Evidence based guidelines for complex regional pain syndrome type 1. *BMC Neurol.* 2010;10:20.

Taylor SS, Noor N, Urits I, Paladini A, Sadhu MS, Gibb C, et al. Complex regional pain syndrome: A comprehensive review. *Pain Ther.* 2021;10:875–892.

12 Children and Burning Pain

David D. Sherry

Case

A 14-year-old girl has severe pain in her right foot and
lower leg. She was playing basketball a month ago
and thinks she may have twisted her ankle. The pain
became progressively worse and she was put in a
splint, which exacerbated her pain. The pain spread
up to below her knee and increased to the point that
she could not tolerate light touch or clothing on her
foot or leg. It hurts too much for her to attend school.
Examination reveals a calm, comfortable girl in no
distress, with normal vital signs. She reports 10/10
pain, which increases with any movement or touching
of her leg from the knee down. Her foot and lower leg
are cool to touch, slightly cyanotic, and edematous.
The allodynia to the lower leg starts approximately
5 cm below the knee when testing from the thigh
down; however, when testing up her leg, allodynia
ends just above the knee. She has minimal active
movement to her ankle and can move her toes. She is
unable to bend her knee. Radiographs are normal.

What Do I Do Now?

PRESENTATION

The case is a typical presentation of a child with complex regional pain syndrome (CRPS). There may or may not be a history of trauma. The lower extremity presentation is much more common in children than in adults. Although there are no validated criteria for CRPS in children, most authors require the presence of at least two autonomic signs such as coolness, cyanosis, edema, or skin changes along with disproportionate pain in the absence of other causes. In addition to disproportionate pain, there is frequently disproportionate disability. These children are unable to go to school or do activities of daily living due to pain. Girls are more frequently affected (80%), as are Caucasians (~90%), and presentation typically occurs in the preteen and early teenage years.[1,2] CRPS has been reported in children as young as 2 years; however, for children under the age of 7 years, the diagnosis should be made with much circumspection. Most authors report that children with CRPS have a particular personality type, including perfectionistic, self-driven, pseudo-mature, accomplished, overly busy, and a pleaser, meeting other's needs to the detriment of their own needs. Rarely are children with CRPS overtly depressed, although depression may be resolved in the pain. Anxiety, however, is not uncommon. Childhood CRPS is part of the spectrum of amplified pain and may coexist with or evolve into other sites of pain or become widespread pain.

The vast majority of children will manifest allodynia, which frequently has a highly variable border when tested repeatedly, as in the child in our case study. A striking feature is the incongruent affect in which the child is calm, interactive, and can be happy and even laughing despite reporting severe pain. Occasionally, children will have hyperbolic pain behaviors, but these generally quickly resolve with distraction. The pain severity frequently increases over time, even if it is present for months to years. The pain is unresponsive to analgesics and other medications typically used for adults with CRPS. These children are at risk of becoming highly overmedicalized, with a prescription given or test ordered for every symptom.[3]

Comorbid conditions include other chronic pain conditions such as irritable bowel syndrome, chest pain, head pain, conversion symptoms (functional neurologic disorder), dysautonomia symptoms (occasionally diagnosed as postural orthostatic tachycardia syndrome), disordered eating, and suicidal ideation. Our patient manifests a conversion symptom by her inability to move her knee even though it was not painful.

Once the diagnosis is clear, it is imperative to validate the pain by letting her know the pain is real and severe. A sympathetically mediated model of pain amplification can tangibly show why the pain is so severe. That is, stimulation of the sympathetic nerves going to the blood vessels lead to ischemia, which causes pain. This ischemic pain then stimulates the sympathetic nerves, leading to more ischemia, and consequently the cyanosis, swelling, and coolness of the extremity. The vicious cycle that is established causes severe, intense pain. The origins for this loop may involve, to varying degrees, trauma, illness, psychological stress, hormones, and genes.

PSYCHODYNAMICS

There is a psycho-pathophysiology in childhood CRPS, and the emotional aspect may play a minor or major role. It is paramount that a psychologist assesses the psychodynamics in all children with CRPS. The psychologist explains the focus of cognitive-behavioral therapy (CBT) and the mind-body connection and introduces coping skills. Before commencing physical and occupational therapy, the child should be deemed emotionally safe, especially if there is a significant emotional trauma history or concern for disordered eating or suicidal ideation. Recommending either a psychologic evaluation or therapy in a way that the child can accept it can be a daunting task. It should be emphasized that a psychologist should be regarded as a teacher or coach. Just as a French teacher helps one learn a language or a soccer coach can help one develop ball-handling skills and strategy, a psychologist is someone who helps one develop skills to better identify and understand the stresses in one's life and deal with these stresses and emotions in constructive ways. Beyond learning coping skills, the child needs to talk about what they do not want to talk about with the psychologist in order to get at deeper core issues.

PHYSICAL AND OCCUPATIONAL THERAPY

Since 1978, the finding that physical and occupational therapy is the mainstay of CRPS treatment has been replicated multiple times.[4] In three subsequent studies, 92% of 191 children responded (most with complete resolution of signs and symptoms).[5-7] There were approximately 30% who experienced a second episode of CRPS, many of whom were able to treat themselves without formal therapy. Of note, the Boston group reported a 42% cure rate using blocks and medications in 1992, but when they converted to more of a physical and occupational therapy approach in 2012, 95% were reported as significantly better.

The amount of therapy varies. It involves explaining that the pain is very real but does not indicate that damage is occurring and that it is important to see what the child can do. Frequently, the child will be able to stand and even take a few steps and do activities reported as impossible. About once or twice a year, at a first visit to the author's clinic, with gentle encouragement, a child will gradually be able to go from crutches to running, and the pain resolves. These can be long-term cures. However, the majority of children will need outpatient physical and occupational therapy because it hurts too much for the child to self-treat. The goal of physical therapy is to increase major motor function and strength, gait training, lower extremity range of motion, aerobic training, and functional activities such as sports or dance. Occupational therapy concentrates on activities of daily living, upper extremity strength and function, and desensitization to the things that exacerbate the pain (touch, bathing, wind, clothing, etc.). The therapists set goals that can be quickly achieved and then advance these goals, making sure the child uses good form without compensating for the pain. This serves to keep the child accountable to the therapist for their home exercise program, thus removing the parents from a therapy role. It is important to not inquire about pain but to assess it nonverbally since the focus is on function, not pain. Likewise, family members should not inquire about pain, and, if the child reports pain, it should be acknowledged but the topic changed to something positive.

STRUCTURED PROGRAMS

If outpatient physical and occupational therapy fails, then the children will need the structure of a program dedicated to CRPS in children. These programs can give 5–6 hours of physical and occupational therapy daily along with the necessary psychologic support, which may be as frequent as daily. Most programs, in addition to a psychologist, have creative arts therapists such as art, music, and dance therapists. Group therapies help establish a community of patients who understand each other's pain and foster wellness.

School issues need to be addressed. School stresses are unique to children who are asked and who often are very self-driven to perform at a high level in a wide range of areas. Adults do not expect themselves to be especially proficient at literature, higher math, history, foreign language, economics, the sciences, geography, drama, dance, and all the other classes these children participate in. Many children feel compelled to take all honors and advanced placement courses.

Most children with CRPS needing intense programs are treated as day hospital patients, although a few are treated in inpatient rehabilitation facilities.

The focus of all physical and occupational therapy is to establish function as quickly as possible. For our patient, this would be removing any aids such as crutches or a cane, generally on the first day of an intense program. Meeting these goals quickly gives a sense of success. Intense desensitization to touch, clothing, and getting a sock and shoe on usually occurs in the first few days. Getting the child to do activities regardless of pain is our goal. The conversion aspects of this child's presentation were purposefully ignored and, as weight-bearing improves, generally so do these symptoms. Conversion symptoms bespeak the need for continuing psychotherapy. The author has seen children resolve all pain and autonomic signs but continue to have conversion symptoms that may take months to years to resolve with psychotherapy while maintaining normal function as much as possible, especially going to school and participating in family activities.

OUTCOMES

Most children who have CRPS have a single episode and seem to do well over time. In one study, 88% had no symptoms after a mean follow-up of 5 years. Importantly, there are children who develop other manifestations of stress, so addressing them at the onset of CRPS is imperative. The author and colleagues have had children develop dysautonomia symptoms, and, one child, thinking there was no hope, died by suicide. Others have developed disordered eating, irritable bowel syndrome, chronic head pain, gender dysmorphia, and new conversion symptoms, including nonepileptic spells, blindness, paralysis, memory issues, and shaking, among other manifestations.

The patient was admitted to our Day Hospital program, which included intense daily physical and occupational therapy program with significant psychological support. After 3 weeks, she regained normal function and resolved all signs and symptoms of CRPS and conversion. She had marked anxiety and school avoidance that were addressed with ongoing psychotherapy.

KEY POINTS TO REMEMBER

- Childhood complex regional pain syndrome (CRPS) is different from that in adults and is on the continuum of amplified pain.
- The mainstay of therapy is physical and occupational therapy focused on function and desensitization of allodynia despite the pain complaint.
- Medications for pain are not indicated and lead to overmedicalization and poorer outcomes.
- Psychological evaluation and therapy are important in treatment and prevention of second episodes or other stress-induced symptoms.

Suggested Reading

Logan DE, Williams SE, Carullo VP, Claar RL, Bruehl S, Berde CB. Children and adolescents with complex regional pain syndrome: More psychologically distressed than other children in pain? *Pain Res Manag.* 2013 Mar-Apr;18(2):87–93.

References
1. Weissmann R, Uziel Y. Pediatric complex regional pain syndrome: A review. *Pediatr Rheumatol Online J.* 2016;14(1):29.
2. Sherry DD. Amplified pain: A helpful diagnosis. *JAMA Pediatr.* 2022 Jan 1;176(1):10–11.
3. Kaufman EL, Tress J, Sherry DD. Trends in medicalization of children with amplified musculoskeletal pain syndrome. *Pain Med.* 2016;18:825–831.

4. Bernstein BH, Singsen BH, Kent JT, Kornreich H, King K, Hicks R, et al. Reflex neurovascular dystrophy in childhood. *J Pediatr*. 1978;93(2):211–215.

5. Sherry DD, Wallace CA, Kelley C, Kidder M, Sapp L. Short- and long-term outcomes of children with complex regional pain syndrome type I treated with exercise therapy. *Clin J Pain*. 1999;15(3):218–223.

6. Brooke V, Janselewitz S. Outcomes of children with complex regional pain syndrome after intensive inpatient rehabilitation. *PM & R*. 2012;4(5):349–354.

7. Logan DE, Carpino EA, Chiang G, Condon M, Firn E, Gaughan VJ, et al. A day-hospital approach to treatment of pediatric complex regional pain syndrome: Initial functional outcomes. *Clin J Pain*. 2012;28(9):766–774.

13 Hope on the Horizon

Oluwatoyin Thompson and Anna Woodbury

Case

A 37-year-old male veteran presents for management
of complex regional pain syndrome (CRPS) pain in the
left foot. He has been followed by a podiatrist for the
past 10 years. He has tried and failed gabapentin and
nonsteroidal anti-inflammatory medications. He has
received oxycodone and hydromorphone as well as
multiple steroid injections to his left foot. He reports
excruciating pain and about 30% reduction in pain
following each steroid injection, which he receives
monthly from his podiatrist. He cannot tolerate air
conditioning or clothing touching the foot and reports
occasional color changes at home; the foot will
occasionally appear purple or bluish. Physical exam
reveals atrophy of the left foot relative to the right and
hair loss over the left lower extremity. He is offered a
lumbar sympathetic plexus block and the possiblity
of spinal cord stimulation, but he is also interested in
complementary, alternative, and adjuvant therapies.

What Do I Do Now?

DIAGNOSIS

Our patient's presentation includes a broad differential ranging from neurologic to cardiogenic to rheumatologic to psychologic pain. Despite a history of rheumatologic abnormalities and some response to steroid injections, complex regional pain syndrome (CRPS) is high on the differential from the patient's history and presentation.

CRPS is a debilitating, painful condition affecting a body region, usually a distal limb, which develops weeks after a preceding injury such as a crush injury, fracture, or surgical operation. Often the pain is accompanied by sensory, vasomotor, sudomotor, motor, and trophic symptoms. Patient presentations are highly variable and can include hyperalgesia, hypesthesia, allodynia, increased/decreased sweating, edema, limited range of motion, muscle weakness, alterations in skin temperature, skin discoloration, and increased/decreased hair or nail growth.

Ideally, CRPS should be recognized in the acute phase because immediate and rapid intervention can prevent its progression to the chronic phase. Unfortunately, in this case, the patient has suffered from inadequately treated CRPS for more than a decade prior to presentation. It is very important for general practitioners and surgeons to recognize CRPS as early as possible to preserve patients' quality of life and prevent disability. Immediate initiation of neuropathic pain medications and referral to an interventional pain specialist for possible sympathetic plexus blocks can prevent disease progression. In addition, adjuvant therapies can help effectively reduce pain.

PATHOGENESIS AND CONSIDERATIONS FOR TREATMENT

Presently the pathogenesis of CRPS is poorly understood; however, there are several hypotheses as to its cause. Autonomic nerve dysfunction likely plays a role in the development of CRPS. One leading theory is that CRPS is caused by central nervous system (CNS) sensitization. In CRPS, the CNS becomes sensitized after a trigger injury that causes an abnormal inflammatory response. Even with an incomplete understanding of the pathogenesis of CRPS, several clinical and adjunct therapies have been developed for the treatment and prevention of CRPS. There are four main pillars in the treatment of CRPS: education, physical rehabilitation, pain management, and psychosocial intervention. The main goals of treatment are to increase limb function, decrease pain, and improve quality of life. Pain management is critical to the treatment of CRPS, and there are many options to choose from. Nonsteroidal anti-inflammatory drugs (NSAIDs), topical creams, antiepileptics, and antidepressants are all options for this patient, and these treatments are discussed further in Chapter 4. Given that this patient has an interest in adjuvant therapies for CRPS, this chapter will focus on the integrative therapies.

AVAILABLE ADJUVANT AND EMERGING THERAPIES

Existing integrative therapies and emerging adjuvant therapies have been shown to decrease pain scores in CRPS. These include manual therapies (acupuncture, massage, chiropractic), energy therapies (reiki, tai chi, acupuncture, yoga), mind-body therapies (yoga, tai chi, mindfulness), nutritional supplements, and noninvasive neuromodulation (emerging), among others. Therapies from each of these broad categories, which at times overlap, are discussed below. A summary of these therapies and their proposed mechanisms can be found in Table 13.1.

Acupuncture

Acupuncture has been increasingly implemented for chronic pain conditions and can be considered as both an energy therapy as well as a manual or manipulative therapy. Acupuncture is a traditional Chinese medicine technique that involves the insertion of needles percutaneously to stimulate acupoints. Acupuncture is thought to modulate the autonomic nervous system and neurohumoral responses to pain, which could have a direct effect for CRPS. A meta-analysis of 36 clinical trials found that acupuncture was more effective than sham and no acupuncture in reducing pain for patients with chronic pain conditions including nonspecific musculoskeletal pain, osteoarthritis, chronic headache, and shoulder pain. In addition, some patients reported a sustained decrease in pain up to a year later.[1] However, a 2013 Cochrane review concluded that there is very low-quality evidence to support that acupuncture treatments are more effective

TABLE 13.1 **Summary of existing and emerging adjuvant therapies for complex regional pain syndrome (CRPS)**

Adjuvant therapy	Description	Proposed mechanism
Acupuncture	Insertion of needles at specific points in the body with the intention of modulating the flow of energy	Activates endogenous opioid system, neuromodulation, and neurohormonal regulation with anti-inflammatory effects
Tai Chi/Qigong	Mindful movement with breathing exercises through a martial art form	Reduces sympathetic outflow, increases endorphin blood levels and neurohormonal regulation with anti-inflammatory effects
Mindfulness meditation	Focusing one's mind on the present moment with openness and without judgement.	Decreases pain anticipation; regulates attention, emotion, perspective, and body awareness
Vitamin C	A water-soluble vitamin found in fruits, vegetables, and supplements	Promotes tendon healing as cofactor in collagen synthesis; antioxidant with anti-inflammatory effects
Transcutaneous electrical nerve stimulation (TENS)	Electrical pulses delivered to the region affected by CRPS	Reduces activity of nociceptors and dorsal horn neurons; increases bodily concentration of endorphins
Noninvasive vagal nerve stimulation (VNS)	Can be delivered via trans-auricular vagus nerve stimulation or trans-cervical vagus nerve stimulation	Modulates the vagus nerve, which may be effective in CRPS given the presence of autonomic dysfunction

Noninvasive brain stimulation	Modalities include repetitive transcranial magnetic stimulation (rTMS), transcranial direct current stimulation (tDCS), and cranial electrotherapy stimulation (CES): rTMS targets deep cortical structures using electromagnetic pulses; tDCS targets superficial cortical structures through direct currents; CES utilizes microampere stimulation to induce alpha waves	Modulates membrane potentials of cortical neural networks, which reduces central nervous system sensitization and CRPS pain
Epidural clonidine	Intrathecal injection or infusion of clonidine	Activates α-2 receptors in the dorsal horn, which decreases pain transmissions
Sympathectomy	Operation that destroys the pathologic portions of the sympathetic chain	Eliminates sympathetic nerves involved in the transmission of dysregulated pain signals in CRPS

than sham in treating CRPS pain.[2] This assessment may be related to the difficulty in adequate sham blinding for acupuncture trials.

Although there is not yet enough research to support or refute the efficacy of acupuncture in CRPS, there are many case reports of acupuncture effectively treating CRPS pain. For example, Hommer et al. reports the use of Chinse Scalp Acupuncture twice per week for 1–4 weeks in two military members with upper extremity CRPS, who, following treatment, experienced sustained functional improvement and normalization of sensation that was still present at 20-month follow-up.[3] Thus, the type of acupuncture may play a role in its efficacy in CRPS. Body acupuncture, ear acupuncture, scalp acupuncture, hand acupuncture, manual acupuncture, and electroacupuncture are all methods of acupuncture delivery.

A particular patient may experience profound pain relief from acupuncture, and it should be considered in the algorithm for personalized pain medicine. The most common adverse events of acupuncture are syncope or soreness, bleeding, bruising, and skin irritation at the site of insertion. The most serious adverse events are pneumothorax and cardiac tamponade from needles inserted too deeply, but this is nearly wholly avoided by booking sessions only with acupuncturists with appropriate training and certification and who are licensed to practice within the state. Nevertheless, acupuncture is generally well-tolerated. Therefore, a trial of two-to-three acupuncture treatments should be considered for interested patients.

Mind-Body Therapies

Mind-body therapies such as yoga and tai chi are low-risk, low-cost interventions that may provide pain relief. Yoga is a Hindu discipline that encompasses breath control, meditation, and specific body postures. Yoga has been adopted into many medical spheres as a form of treatment. One study found that yoga improved occupational performance, increased activity enjoyment, and decreased depression in patients with chronic pain.[4] Tai chi is a Chinese martial art consisting of movement-based meditation as the body slowly assumes specific poses. Qigong is a system of calisthenics similar to tai chi, but whereas tai chi focuses on movement that encompasses the entire body, qigong focuses on one particular body movement at a time. A Cochrane review found very low-quality evidence that qigong is more effective than sham therapy in reducing CRPS pain, mostly due to the limited number of high-quality clinical trials available.[2] Mind-body therapies are a type of exercise with minimal risk; the positions and physical strain of these activities can be adjusted for a patient's comfort level and can benefit self-management of pain as well as desensitization.

Relaxation-based mind-body techniques such as deep breathing and meditation are generally safe, with virtually no adverse events. Deep breathing therapy is a technique in which patients breathe with their core. Breathing techniques can be accompanied by imagery, progressive muscle relaxation, and/or meditation. Meditation has several benefits such as stress reduction, increased attentiveness, and improved mood. A meta-analysis concluded that mindfulness meditation decreases pain and improves quality of life in patients suffering from chronic pain.[5]

Nutritional Approaches

Nutritional supplements encompass a wide range of herbs, vitamins, and food and will only be briefly touched on here. Many herbs and supplements reduce inflammation such as turmeric, ginger, nutmeg, and cinnamon, or alleviate pain, such as cannabis and magnesium. In addition, vitamin C has been studied specifically in the prevention of CRPS. A meta-analysis found that a daily dose of vitamin C after an injury and/or surgery reduced the prevalence of CRPS type I as compared to placebo.[6] Patients, especially those undergoing high-risk distal limb operations, should take 500 mg of vitamin C daily for 50 days following surgery or injury to prevent the development of CRPS.

Neuromodulation/Electrical Stimulation

Several emerging therapies utilize neuromodulation, including noninvasive electrical stimulation devices and new rehabilitative techniques. Prism adaptation therapy (PAT) is one such rehabilitative technique in which a patient wears optical prisms while undergoing 20-minute visuo-motor training sessions. A standard treatment course is 10 sessions over 2 weeks. PAT has been shown to help spatial neglect in right-brain stroke patients because it improves their functional behaviors like getting dressed.[7] Another hypothesis regarding the pathogenies of CRPS is that the pain is caused by an abnormal cognitive perception and/or representation of the affected limb. Therefore, PAT could be an effective treatment. Several small studies have shown that PAT visual displacement training *away* from the affected limb reduces CRPS pain.[8]

For patients who are comfortable with noninvasive electrotherapeutic device treatments, consider transcutaneous electrical nerve stimulation (TENS), pulsed electromagnetic field therapy (PEMF), or noninvasive vagal nerve stimulation (VNS). TENS is an inexpensive self-administrated peripheral stimulation device that works by delivering electrical pulses to nociceptors through electrodes on the affected skin. TENS has been shown to reduce neuropathic pain.[9] TENS is very safe, with its most common side effect being skin irritation at the site of the electrodes. Some patients do report nausea or feeling faint after sessions. TENS has been associated with seizures, but this side effect is very rare. There is also the risk of burn injury but only if TENS is used for prolonged periods of time. TENS should be used in caution in patients who have pacemakers, who may be pregnant, and/or who have a history of epilepsy. Another safe, inexpensive noninvasive device is PEMF. During a PEMF session, a patient lies down next to a device that generates pulsed electromagnetic fields with varied intensity, waveforms, and frequencies.

Another transcutaneous device that works through a different mechanism is noninvasive VNS, which utilizes a device placed on the ear or neck that stimulates the vagus nerve through skin electrodes. Stimulating the vagus nerve induces the cholinergic anti-inflammatory pathway and reduces nociception. Noninvasive VNS is a promising treatment since it targets CRPS's autonomic dysfunction by stimulating parasympathetics and abnormal inflammation through the cholinergic anti-inflammatory pathways.[10]

Another class of adjuvant and emerging therapies involves noninvasive brain stimulation such as repetitive transcranial magnetic stimulation (rTMS), transcranial direct current stimulation (tDCS), and cranial electrotherapy stimulation (CES). rTMS involves an electromagnetic coil placed against a patient's scalp to deliver repetitive electromagnetic pulses through the skull to stimulate the deep cortical structures of the brain. rTMS has been approved by the US Food and Drug Administration (FDA) for the treatment of refractory depression, obsessive compulsive disorder, and smoking cessation. Current studies are evaluating whether rTMS could also be effective for treating chronic pain and CRPS. However, according to a 2013 Cochrane review, there have not been enough studies to support or refute its effectiveness.[2] The sessions are typically painless, with mild side effects such as headaches or feeling faint. However, adverse events such as seizures and hearing loss can occur if the proper protective measures are not taken. rTMS is contraindicated in persons with any metal head, neck, or ear implants.

tDCS is another noninvasive brain stimulation treatment, and devices can be easily acquired online through direct-to-consumer websites without a prescription. A low-intensity direct electric current passes continuously between two electrodes placed on a patient's head. The direct current modulates neuronal activity in the superficial cortical structures of the brain. Several small studies have reported that tDCS alleviates pain in neuropathic chronic pain conditions.[11] tDCS is inexpensive, portable, and relatively safe. The most common side effects are skin irritation or burns under the electrodes. tDCS should be used in caution in patients with a history of seizures and in patients with head and neck bone or skin lesions. tDCS should not be used on patients with head implants or tumors.

Finally, CES is a noninvasive approach to chronic pain that involves stimulation via clips placed on the ear lobe. Its mechanism is not well-described, but devices are typically compact and can also be purchased without a doctor's prescription. Alpha-stim is one device utilized to deliver CES that is FDA-cleared and has been shown to have positive effects in anxiety, insomnia, depression, and pain management.

OPTIONS IN TREATMENT-RESISTANT COMPLEX REGIONAL PAIN SYNDROME

If a patient fails all standard and adjuvant treatments, epidural clonidine or sympathectomy can be considered as alternate emerging therapies.

Clonidine, an α-2-agonist, can be injected or infused into a patient's epidural space through a spinal catheter. The catheter is inserted in the cervical spine for upper extremity pathology and into the lumbar spine for lower extremity pathology. The procedure is very effective for pain relief, but its adverse effects include sedation, hypotension, and bradycardia.[12] Therefore, patients need to be carefully monitored during and after the procedure.

Sympathectomy is a minimally invasive procedure in which portions of the sympathetic chain are cauterized or chemically destroyed. Sympathectomy may reduce CRPS pain but should only be performed in patients who have had positive responses to nerve blocks. A 2010 Cochrane review concluded that there is very weak evidence for sympathectomy in improving CRPS pain.[13] In addition, sympathectomy has serious side effects such as hypotension and bradycardia. It also has serious adverse event risks such as increased pain, new neuropathic pain, erratic sweating, and Horner's syndrome.[13]

Due to severe potential complications and side effects associated with epidural clonidine and sympathectomy, either treatment could pose too great a risk for a patient. The risks and benefits should be discussed extensively with a patient before undergoing either procedure. While these treatments are available, they are not considered first line.

CASE (CONTINUED)

The patient was first instructed on mindfulness meditation, a relaxation-based mind-body technique for pain. He was encouraged to perform it every day and was given a list of applications and websites that offer guided meditations. He was also scheduled for electroacupuncture two times a week for 4 weeks, to be followed by maintenance acupuncture once per month. By Week 3, he reported a 2-point reduction in his left foot pain score. His left foot still appeared atrophic compared to his right, but he was more comfortable wearing shoes and having clothing or air touch his foot. Given the partial relief from his acupuncture sessions, he was able to discontinue steroid injections. However, he still wished to decrease the need for opioid analgesics. Therefore, he was scheduled for a lumbar sympathetic plexus block. He reported 80% relief following each block, but the relief dissipated after 48 hours. Therefore, he was offered a spinal cord stimulator trial and eventually underwent a spinal cord stimulator implant procedure. He was able to return to work and cease all opioid analgesics following implantation. He continued to use mindfulness meditation and acupuncture to manage his other pain conditions, which included gout and postherpetic neuralgia.

SUMMARY

Although many of the adjuvant and emerging treatments listed do not yet have large studies for their efficacy in CRPS, these treatment options should be considered for their potential to provide increased pain relief. One of these adjuvant treatments could be pivotal in managing an individual's pain. If a patient's pain is not improving, or if a patient would like to try adjuvant treatments, it is important to discuss with them the risks and benefits of all available therapies. The discussed therapies, especially those that are minimally invasive and low risk, should be initiated early in the treatment algorithm and can be used as an adjunct or complement to conventional therapies.

KEY POINTS TO REMEMBER

- It is important to recognize and diagnosis complex regional pain syndrome (CRPS) early.
- A trial of low-risk therapies such as meditation, yoga, tai chi, and acupuncture should be provided to all willing patients without contraindications.
- Patients should take 500 mg of vitamin C daily for 50 days following distal limb surgery or injury to prevent the development of CRPS.
- Several safe, inexpensive, and portable devices can be used to alleviate CRPS pain.
- Emerging therapies such as epidural clonidine and sympathectomy have severe risks and side effects that must be carefully discussed with all patients considering these therapies.

Suggested Reading

Moisset X, Lanteri-Minet M, Fontaine D. Neurostimulation methods in the treatment of chronic pain. *J Neural Transm*. 2020;127:673–686. https://doi.org/10.1007/s00 702-019-02092-y

O'Connell NE, Wand BM, McAuley JH, Marston L, Moseley GL. Interventions for treating pain and disability in adults with complex regional pain syndrome: An overview of systematic reviews. *Cochrane Database Syst Rev.* 2013;4:CD009416. doi:10.1002/14651858.CD009416.pub2.

Urits I, Schwartz RH, Orhurhu V, Maganty NV, Reilly BT, Patel PM, et al. A comprehensive review of alternative therapies for the management of chronic pain patients: Acupuncture, tai chi, osteopathic manipulative medicine, and chiropractic care. *Adv Ther.* 2021 Jan;38(1):76–89. doi:10.1007/s12325-020-01554-0. Epub 2020 Nov 12. PMID: 33184777; PMCID: PMC7854390.

Vickers AJ, Vertosick EA, Lewith G, MacPherson H, Foster NE, Sherman KJ, et al.; Acupuncture Trialists' Collaboration. Acupuncture for chronic pain: Update of an individual patient data meta-analysis. *J Pain.* 2018 May;19(5):455–474. doi:10.1016/j.jpain.2017.11.005. Epub 2017 Dec 2. PMID: 29198932; PMCID: PMC5927830.

References

1. Vickers AJ, Vertosick EA, Lewith G, MacPherson H, Foster NE, Sherman KJ, et al.; Acupuncture Trialists' Collaboration. Acupuncture for chronic pain: Update of an individual patient data meta-analysis. *J Pain.* 2018 May;19(5):455–474. doi:10.1016/j.jpain.2017.11.005. Epub 2017 Dec 2. PMID: 29198932; PMCID: PMC5927830.

2. O'Connell NE, Wand BM, McAuley JH, Marston L, Moseley GL. Interventions for treating pain and disability in adults with complex regional pain syndrome: An overview of systematic reviews. *Cochrane Database SystRev.* 2013;4:CD009416. doi:10.1002/14651858.CD009416.pub2

3. Hommer DH. Chinese scalp acupuncture relieves pain and restores function in complex regional pain syndrome. *Mil Med.* 2012 Oct;177(10):1231–1234. doi:10.7205/milmed-d-12-00193. PMID: 23113454.

4. Schmid AA, Van Puymbroeck M, Fruhauf CA, Bair MJ, Portz JD. Yoga improves occupational performance, depression, and daily activities for people with chronic pain. *Work.* 2019;63(2):181–189. doi:10.3233/WOR-192919. PMID: 31156199.

5. Hilton L, Hempel S, Ewing BA, Apaydin E, Xenakis L, Newberry S, et al. Mindfulness meditation for chronic pain: Systematic review and meta-analysis. *Ann Behav Med.* 2017 Apr;51(2):199–213. doi:10.1007/s12160-016-9844-2. PMID: 27658913; PMCID: PMC5368208.

6. Seth I, Bulloch G, Seth N, Siu A, Clayton S, Lower K, et al. Effect of perioperative vitamin c on the incidence of complex regional pain syndrome: A systematic review and meta-analysis. *J Foot Ankle Surg.* 2022 Jul-Aug;61(4):748–754. doi:10.1053/j.jfas.2021.11.008. Epub 2021 Nov 21. PMID: 34961681.

7. Goedert KM, Zhang JY, Barrett AM. Prism adaptation and spatial neglect: The need for dose-finding studies. *Front Hum Neurosci.* 2015 Apr 30;9:243. doi:10.3389/fnhum.2015.00243. PMID: 25983688; PMCID: PMC4415396.

8. Sumitani M, Rossetti Y, Shibata M, Matsuda Y, Sakaue G, Inoue T, et al. Prism adaptation to optical deviation alleviates pathologic pain. *Neurology*. 2007;68(2), 128–133. https://doi.org/10.1212/01.wnl.0000250242.99683.57

9. Gibson W, Wand BM, O'Connell NE. Transcutaneous electrical nerve stimulation (TENS) for neuropathic pain in adults. *Cochrane Database Syst*. 2017;9:CD011976. https://doi.org/10.1002/14651858.CD011976.pub2

10. Baronio M, Sadia H, Paolacci S, Prestamburgo D, Miotti D, Guardamagna VA, et al. Molecular aspects of regional pain syndrome. *Pain Res Manag*. 2020 Apr 11;2020:7697214. doi:10.1155/2020/7697214. PMID: 32351641; PMCID: PMC7171689.

11. Lefaucheur J-P. A comprehensive database of published tDCS clinical trials (2005–2016). *Neurophysiol Clin*. 2016;46:319–398. https://doi.org/10.1016/j.neucli.2016.10.002

12. Rauck RL, Eisenach JC, Jackson K, Young LD, Southern J. Epidural clonidine treatment for refractory reflex sympathetic dystrophy. *Anesthesiology*. 1993 Dec;79(6):1163–1169; discussion 27A. PMID: 8267190.

13. Straube S, Derry S, Moore RA, McQuay HJ. Cervico-thoracic or lumbar sympathectomy for neuropathic pain and complex regional pain syndrome. *Cochrane Database Syst Rev*. 2010 Jul 7;(7):CD002918. doi:10.1002/14651858. CD002918.pub2. Update in: *Cochrane Database Syst Rev*. 2013;9:CD002918. PMID: 20614432; PMCID: PMC4053682.

Index

For the benefit of digital users, indexed terms that span two pages (e.g., 52–53) may, on occasion, appear on only one of those pages.

Page references followed by *t* denote tables.

Chinese Scalp Acupuncture, 114
chiropractic care, 120
chronic CRPS
    pathophysiology of, 23
    standard approach to, 36
clinical cases, 1, 11, 19, 27, 47, 55, 63, 68,
        71, 77, 85, 95, 101, 109, 118
clodronate, 34
clonidine
    epidural, 112t, 117, 118, 119
    ketamine infusion therapy with, 79
    nerve blocks with, 96, 97
cognitive-behavioral therapy (CBT), 38–
        39, 103
contiguous spread of CRPS, 86
contralateral or "mirror image" spread, 86,
        87, 88–89
conversion symptoms, 102–3
corticosteroids, 33, 97
COVID vaccination, 1, 5–6
cranial electrotherapy stimulation (CES),
        112t, 116–17
C-reactive protein (CRP), 14–15
CT scans, 14

deep breathing, 115
deep venous thrombosis (DVT), 15–16
depression, 4, 32, 37, 39, 102
desensitization, 89
dexamethasone, 50
diagnosis, 12–14, 17, 110
    Budapest Consensus Criteria, 12,
        13t, 17, 28
    early, 74
    standard approach, 28
diagonal spread of CRPS, 87
differential diagnosis, 14–17
dimethyl sulfoxide (DMSO), 33–34
distal radius fractures, 97
dorsal root ganglion (DRG) stimulation
    adjustability, 67
    clinical case, 68
    complications, 67–68
    costs, 67

efficacy, 65–66
    implantation site, 65
    learning curve with, 67
    long-term efficacy, 67
    mechanism of action, 64
    patient selection for, 65, 67
    pros and cons, 66–67
    vs. spinal cord stimulation (SCS), 64–
        65, 68
    targeted area, 64
duloxetine, 35, 38–39
dural puncture, 59
dysautonomia, 102–3

electroacupuncture, 118
electrotherapy, 29, 112t, 115–17
emerging therapies, 111–17, 112t, 119
    clinical cases, 118
    for treatment-resistant CRPS, 117–18
energy therapy, 111
epidemiology, 2, 6, 7
epidural block, 51, 96
epidural hematoma, 59
erythrocyte sedimentation rate (ESR), 14–15
erythromelalgia, 16
European Federation of Neurological
        Societies, 58
exercise, therapeutic, 29, 30–31
exposure therapy, graded (GEXP), 29–30

factitious disorders, 17
failed back surgery syndrome, 57
Fear Avoidance Hierarchy, 30–31
femoral nerve block, 97
fibromyalgia, 86, 95
fractures, 2, 95, 97
free radical scavengers, 32–34
functional limitations, 39–40
functional magnetic resonance imaging
        (fMRI), 22

gabapentin, 32
gate control theory, 36, 56–57
genetic factors, 21t, 23, 24

manual therapy, 29, 30–31, 111, 120

medical conditions, 3–4

medical therapy, 31–35

medications. *See* pharmacotherapy; *specific medications*

meditation, 112*t*, 115, 118, 119

mental health conditions, 37

midazolam, 79

migraine, 3–4, 6

mind-body therapy, 111, 114–15

mindfulness meditation, 112*t*, 118

"mirror image" spread, 86, 87, 88–89

mirror therapy
    for spread of CRPS, 89
    standard approach, 29–30

monitoring medications, 39

morphine, 66, 97

multimodal therapy
    with interventional treatments, 48
    for spread of CRPS, 89
    standard approach, 39

N-acetylcysteine (NAC), 33–34

neridronate, 34

nerve blocks, 14
    clinical cases, 118
    perioperative, 96, 97
    peripheral, 51, 53
    sympathetic, 14, 48–51, 53

neurogenic inflammation, 20

neuromodulation, 64–65, 72, 111, 115–17. *See also* dorsal root ganglion (DRG) stimulation; peripheral nerve stimulation (PNS); spinal cord stimulation (SCS)
    for spread of CRPS, 90

neuropeptide Y, 20, 21*t*

N-methyl-D-aspartate (NMDA) receptor antagonists, 48

nociplastic pain, 36

nonsteroidal anti-inflammatory drugs (NSAIDs), 110–11
    and risk of CRPS, 3–4

standard approach, 32–33
    topical, 35

nortriptyline, 38–39

nutritional supplements, 111, 115

obesity, 81

occupational therapy (OT)
    for childhood CRPS, 103–4, 106
    for spread of CRPS, 89
    standard approach, 30–31, 38–39

ondansetron, 79

opioids, 35, 66

orthopedic surgery, 98

pain
    behavioral-psycho-social component, 17
    chronic, 36
    conceptualization of, 36
    definition of, 36
    gate control theory of, 36, 56–57
    nociplastic, 36
    patient education about, 29, 40
    sympathetically independent (SIP), 48–49, 51, 53
    sympathetically mediated (SMP), 48, 51–52, 53

pain neuroscience education, 29

pain psychology, 35–38

pain relief, 110–11. *See also* management
    with dorsal root ganglion (DRG) stimulation, 64–67
    with spinal cord stimulation (SCS), 56, 64–65
    targeted, 66

pamidronate, 34

paralysis, 59

parecoxib, 33

paresthesia, 64, 67

pathogenesis, 18, 20, 21*t*, 23, 110–11

pathophysiology, 20–24, 21*t*, 25, 72–73

patient education, 29, 40, 110–11

pediatric patients. *See* childhood CRPS

perioperative treatment, 96

spread of CRPS (*cont.*)
   independent, 87
   ipsilateral, 87, 89
   management of, 89–90
   pathogenesis of, 88–89
   pattern types, 86–87
   predisposing factors, 87
   typical characteristics, 87–88
stellate ganglion block (SGB), 49–50, 53
steroids, 89
substance P, 20, 21*t*, 22
subtypes of CRPS, 12
surgery
   inciting events, 2, 90
   prevention of postsurgical CRPS, 96–97,
      98, 115, 119
   for spread of CRPS, 90
sympathectomy, 112*t*, 117, 118
   clinical case, 118
sympathetically independent pain (SIP),
      48–49, 51, 53
sympathetically mediated pain (SMP), 48,
      51–52, 53
sympathetic nerve blocks, 14, 48–51, 53
sympathetic nervous system, 21*t*, 22–23

Tai Chi, 112*t*, 114–15, 119, 120
thoracic outlet syndrome (TOC), 16
thoracic sympathetic block, 49–50, 53
topical therapy, 35, 110–11
total knee arthroplasty, 96–97
tramadol, 35, 38–39
transcranial direct current stimulation
      (tDCS), 112*t*, 116–17
transcranial magnetic stimulation, repetitive
      (rTMS), 112*t*, 116–17
transcutaneous electrical nerve stimulation
      (TENS), 29, 112*t*, 116
treatment. *See also* management
   adjuvant therapy, 35, 97, 111–17,
      112*t*, 118–19
   early, 74

emerging therapies, 110–19, 112*t*
interventional, 48
perioperative, 96
rehabilitation approaches, 29–30
therapeutic exercise, 29, 30–31
treatment plans, 39
treatment-resistant CRPS, 72
   alternate emerging therapies for, 117–18
   Bier block for, 52
   neuromodulation for, 64–65
tricyclic antidepressants (TCAs), 32,
      35, 39
tumor necrosis factor (TNF)-α, 20, 21*t*
type I CRPS, 12
   clinical cases, 47, 63
   after COVID-19 vaccination, 5–6
   pathophysiology, 23
   prevalence, 2
   SCS treatment of, 57–58, 60
   spread of, 91
type II CRPS, 2, 12

upper extremity CRPS, 66
upper thoracic sympathetic block, 49–
      50, 53
US Drug Enforcement Agency (DEA), 78
US Food and Drug Administration (FDA),
      32, 116–17

vaccination, 5–6
vagal nerve stimulation (VNS), noninvasive,
      112*t*, 116
vascular disorders, 15–16
virtual reality, 29
vitamin C, 96, 97, 98
   postoperative, 115, 119
   summary, 112*t*

warm CRPS, 20
white blood cell (WBC) count, 14–15

yoga, 114–15, 119